Supplement 4 zu Band 23, April 2000

Offizielles Organ der Deutschen Gesellschaft für Hämatologie und Onkologie,
der Österreichischen Gesellschaft für Hämatologie und Onkologie,
der Österreichischen Krebsgesellschaft – Krebsliga unter Fortführung der
«Österreichischen Zeitung für Onkologie»

ONKOLOGIE

• International Journal for Cancer Research and Treatment

KARGER

Basel · Freiburg · Paris · London · New York ·
New Delhi · Bangkok · Singapore · Tokyo · Sydney

Bibliographische Dienste
Biological Abstracts
Current Contents/Clinical Medicine
Excerpta Medica/EMBASE
Medical Documentation Service
Reference Update
Research Alert
Science Citation Index
SCISEARCH Database

S. Karger · Medical and Scientific Publishers · Basel · Freiburg · Paris · London · New York · New Delhi · Bangkok · Singapore · Tokyo · Sydney

Die Zeitschrift erscheint zweimonatlich; pro Jahr erscheint 1 Band zu je 6 Heften. Bezugspreis für Jahrgang 23, 2000, DEM 218,– / CHF 170,–, einschließlich MwSt., zuzüglich Postgebühren. Der Abonnementpreis ist im voraus zahlbar. Das Abonnement der Zeitschrift läuft weiter, wenn es nicht spätestens 4 Wochen vor Abschluß eines Bandes abbestellt wird.
Abonnementbestellungen können bei jeder Buchhandlung oder direkt beim Verlag aufgegeben werden:
Deutschland: S. Karger GmbH, Lörracher Str. 16a, D-79115 Freiburg, Telefon +49 7 61 45 20 70, Telefax +49 7 61 4 52 07 14, E-mail Information@Karger.de, Postbank München 400 80-807.
Übrige Länder: S. Karger AG, Allschwilerstr. 10, Postfach, CH-4009 Basel, Telefon +41 61 3 06 11 11, Telefax +41 61 3 06 12 34, E-mail Karger@Karger.ch.

Anzeigen: S. Karger Verlag für Medizin und Naturwissenschaften GmbH, Lörracher Str. 16a, D-79115 Freiburg, Telefon +49 7 61 45 20 70.
Gültig ist die Preisliste Nr. 10 vom 1. Januar 1999.

Supplement 4 zu Band 23, April 2000; ISBN 3-8055-7089-9

Verlagsleitung und presserechtlich verantwortlich: Sibylle Hopf
Anzeigenleitung: Susanne Meister
Produktionsleitung: Georg Brunner

Herstellung: Konkordia Druck GmbH, Eisenbahnstraße 31, D-77815 Bühl

KARGER

Fax +49 761 4 52 07 14
E-mail Information@Karger.de
www.karger.com

Home Page der Zeitschrift:
www.karger.com/journals/onk

ONKOLOGIE

Supplement 4 zu Band 23,
April 2000

Irinotecan (Campto®)

Clinical Overview

Guest Editor
D. K. Hossfeld, Hamburg

KARGER

Basel · Freiburg · Paris · London · New York ·
New Delhi · Bangkok · Singapore · Tokyo · Sydney

Contents · Inhalt

ONKOLOGIE

Vol. 23, Suppl 4, April 2000

KARGER

Fax +49 761 4 52 07 14
E-mail Information@Karger.de
www.karger.com

Artikel (Volltext) und Inhaltsverzeichnisse
sowie das vorläufige Inhaltsverzeichnis des nächsten Heftes:
www.karger.com/journals/onk/onk_bk.htm

ONKOLOGIE

Onkologie 2000;23(suppl 4):1

Editorial

Within the past few years, irinotecan (CPT-11, Campto®), a new topoisomerase I inhibitor, has proved to be an effective drug for treatment of colorectal carcinomas and a growing number of other tumor entities.

Two randomized studies on second-line treatment of colorectal cancer have shown that chemotherapy with irinotecan alone every 3 weeks was significantly superior to the 'best supportive care' and best possible 5-fluorouracil treatment regimens with respect to overall survival. As a result, the German health administration authorized irinotecan for use in this indication in 1998.

The combination of irinotecan and 5-fluorouracil/folinic acid has also been used for primary treatment of metastatic colorectal cancer since 1997. Weekly (AIO regimen) and biweekly regimens (De Gramont regimen) have been investigated. A European multicenter study demonstrated the superiority of combination chemotherapy with irinotecan plus 5-fluorouracil/folinic acid to treatment with 5-fluorouracil/folinic acid alone [1]. The combination was superior with respect to the response rate, the time to tumor progression, and overall survival. This was the first combination chemotherapy for primary treatment of patients with colorectal cancer that achieved better overall survival rates than the current standard therapy. The European results were confirmed in an American study in which combination chemotherapy with irinotecan plus 5-fluorouracil/folinic acid (bolus therapy) achieved better response rates and survival rates than monotherapy with 5-fluorouracil/folinic acid alone (bolus therapy according to the Mayo Clinic protocol) or with irinotecan alone. These findings were first presented by Saltz and co-workers at the meeting of the American Society of Clinical Oncology in Atlanta in 1999.

In light of the positive results of these randomized multicenter trials on primary treatment of colorectal cancer, irinotecan was combined with 5-fluorouracil/folinic acid and other cytostatic agents to treat other tumor entities (gastric, biliary, cervical, lung, and ovarian cancer) and has already been assessed in a number of studies.

The goal of this supplement is to provide an overview of irinotecan applications. It contains summaries of completed studies and a survey of currently ongoing clinical trials of irinotecan in various tumor entities and indications.

D. K. Hossfeld, Hamburg

References

1 Douillard JY, et al: Irinotecan combined with fluorouracil compared with fluorouracil alone as first-line treatment for metastatic colorectal cancer: A multicentre randomised trial. Lancet 2000;355:1041–1047.

KARGER

Fax +49 761 4 52 07 14
E-mail Information@Karger.de
www.karger.com

Accessible online at:
www.karger.com/journals/onk

Prof. Dr. D.K. Hossfeld
Universitätskrankenhaus Eppendorf
Abt. Onkologie und Hämatologie
Martinistraße 52
D-20246 Hamburg (Germany)

ONKOLOGIE

Onkologie 2000;23(suppl 4):2–7

Preclinical Evaluation of Irinotecan

U. Vanhoefer[a] W. Achterrath[b] H. Wilke[a] S. Seeber[a]

[a]Department of Internal Medicine (Cancer Research), West German Cancer Center, University of Essen Medical School,
[b]Aventis Pharma, Department of Clinical Research, Oncology, Bad Soden

Key Words
Irinotecan · CPT-11 · Preclinical evaluation

Summary
DNA topoisomerase I (TOP-I) is a ubiquitous nuclear enzyme, which plays a key role in cellular processes like DNA replication and transcription. With the realization that TOP-I is an important target in cancer therapy, TOP-I interactive agents entered intensive preclinical and clinical evaluation programs. Irinotecan is enzymatically converted by carboxylesterase to its most active cytotoxic metabolite 7-ethyl-10-hydroxy-camptothecin (SN-38), which is inactivated by hepatic biotransformation in a sequential metabolism. SN-38 establishes an equilibrium between the pharmacologically active closed lactone ring and the inactive hydroxy acid form by reversible pH-dependent hydrolysis. SN-38 exerts its cytotoxic mechanism by generating intermediate forms of drug-stabilized covalent DNA/TOP-I complexes, which may lead by collision with the moving replication complexes to arrest and disassembly of the replication machinery. In preclinical models, acquired resistance to camptothecin derivatives has been mainly related to down-regulation of TOP-I expression as well as to alterations in structure and function of the TOP-I gene. Based on promising preclinical data on synergistic cytotoxic drug interactions, a variety of irinotecan-based combinations are currently under clinical evaluation (e.g., cisplatin, oxaliplatin, raltitrexed, taxanes). The task of future investigations will be to identify molecular markers, which are predictive for tumor response to irinotecan-based chemotherapy.

Schlüsselwörter
Irinotecan · CPT-11 · Präklinische Evaluation

Zusammenfassung
Die DNA-Topoisomerase-I (TOP-I) ist ein zelluläres Enzym mit einer Schlüsselrolle in der DNA-Replikation und Transkription. Mit der Erkenntnis, daß TOP-I für die Wirkung der Zytostatikatherapie von besonderer Bedeutung ist, wurden TOP-I-interaktive Substanzen einer intensiven präklinischen und klinischen Evaluierung unterzogen. Irinotecan wird enzymatisch über die Carboxylesterase zellulär zum aktiven zytotoxischen Metaboliten 7-Ethyl-10-Hydroxycamptothecin (SN-38) umgewandelt. Die Inaktivierung von SN-38 erfolgt mittels einer sequentiellen hepatischen Biotransformation. SN-38 bildet über eine pH-abhängige Hydrolyse ein Gleichgewicht zwischen der pharmakologisch aktiven geschlossenen Ringform und der inaktiven Hydroxyform. Die Zytotoxizität von Irinotecan korreliert mit der Bildung von SN-38-stabilisierten DNA/TOP-I Komplexen, die während der S-Phase mit der DNA-Replikationsmaschinerie interferieren und zu deren Instabilität führen. Die Resistenz gegenüber Camptothecinderivaten wurde in präklinischen Modellen haupt-sächlich mit einer verminderten TOP-I-Expression, sowie mit Änderungen in der Enzymstruktur und Funktion in Zusammenhang gebracht. Synergistische zytotoxische Interaktionen von Irinotecan mit einer Vielzahl anderer Zytostatika führten zu einer intensiven klinischen Evaluierung dieser Kombinationschemotherapien (z.B. Fluoropyrimidine, Oxaliplatin, Cisplatin, Raltitrexed, Taxane). Das Ziel künftiger Untersuchungen wird die Identifizierung molekularer Marker sein, die eine prädiktive Aussage über das Ansprechen auf Chemotherapie mit Irinotecan erlauben.

KARGER

Fax +49 761 4 52 07 14
E-mail Information@Karger.de
www.karger.com

Accessible online at:
www.karger.com/journals/onk

U. Vanhoefer
Department of Internal Medicine (Cancer Research),
West German Cancer Center, University of Essen Medical School,
D-45122 Essen (Germany)
Tel. +49-201723-2012, Fax -5736
E-mail udo.vanhoefer@uni-essen.de

Introduction

Irinotecan (7-ethyl-10-[4(-1-piperidino)-1-piperidino] carbonyloxy camptothecin) is a new semisynthetic derivative of the natural alkaloid camptothecin, with a new mechanism of cytotoxic action by converting topoisomerase I into a lethal agent [1–4]. Preclinical and clinical studies with irinotecan demonstrated a broad spectrum of therapeutic activity against solid tumors [5–7]. Of special interest was the demonstration of considerable activity against 5-fluorouracil (5-FU) refractory colorectal cancer, leading to a comprehensive evaluation program of irinotecan as single agent and as part of combination therapies in advanced colorectal cancer. The results of these studies established irinotecan as one of the most active drugs in the treatment of advanced colorectal cancer [8–15].

The present article describes the mechanism of cytotoxicity of irinotecan with special emphasis on drug resistance and drug interactions.

Topoisomerase I

DNA topoisomerase I (TOP-I) is a ubiquitous nuclear enzyme with key roles in DNA replication, transcription, and possibly DNA recombination and repair [1, 3, 16, 17]. TOP-I relaxes torsionally strained supercoiled duplex DNA by covalently linking its tyrosine hydroxyl group at position 723 to the 3'-phosphate at the DNA break site, which results in an enzyme-linked single-strand nick in the phosphodiester backbone of the DNA. This enzyme-bridged single-strand DNA break allows the intact DNA strand to pass through. After rotation of the intact DNA strand, DNA religation is initiated [16, 18–20]. Human TOP-I mRNA transcription and protein expression is regulated by a complex system of negative and positive transcription factors [21–29]. Recent data suggest that the phosphorylation state of TOP-I is one of the key mechanisms of post-translational regulation, involving protein kinase C and casein II-associated tyrosine kinase [30–32].

Mechanisms of Cytotoxic Action

Irinotecan belongs to a new class of antineoplastic agents, called topoisomerase-I interactive compounds, which share a common new mechanism of cytotoxic action by converting topoisomerase I into a cytotoxic agent [1–4].

In vivo, irinotecan is enzymatically converted by carboxylesterase to its most active cytotoxic metabolite 7-ethyl-10-hydroxy-camptothecin (SN-38) [2, 4, 33, 34]. SN-38 establishes an equilibrium between the pharmacologically active closed lactone ring and the inactive open ring hydroxy acid form by reversible pH-dependent hydrolysis [34]. SN-38 is referred to as a topoisomerase-I interactive agent, that exerts its cytotoxic activity by generating intermediate forms of drug-stabilized covalent DNA/TOP-I complexes, referred to as cleavable complexes. The collision of these drug-stabilized enzyme-bridged DNA breaks with the moving replication machinery may lead to cell death due to replication arrest and replication fork disassembly [1, 35–41]. An important feature in terms of mechanism of action is that SN-38 exerts its cytotoxicity by trapping cleavable complexes rather than by inhibition of TOP-I enzyme function. Recent studies suggest that camptothecin derivatives trap TOP-I predominantly in actively transcribed genes [42, 43]. In addition, in vitro and in vivo studies indicate that prolonged exposure to irinotecan may enhance antitumor activity [44, 45].

Studies on cell cultures suggest that TOP-I expression may predict tumor response to camptothecin derivatives [46–48]. Of importance is that increased TOP-I expression was found in human tumor samples, especially for colon cancer when compared to normal colon mucosa [49–51]. However, evaluation of cell lines and tumor samples revealed that interindividual TOP-I expression varies widely [52–54]. There is evidence that the induction of TOP-I cleavable complexes may be a better response predictor than TOP-I expression alone [55]. In addition, human tumor carboxylesterase activity has been correlated with cytotoxicity of irinotecan [56]. Furthermore, mutations of the TOP-I gene appear not to contribute to clinical resistance to camptothecins and no correlation was found between TOP-I expression in human biopsy samples and clinical resistance to irinotecan or topotecan [52, 57].

In preclinical models, acquired resistance to TOP-I interactive drugs has been related to down-regulation of TOP-I expression as well as to alterations in TOP-I gene structure and function (e.g., point mutations, deletions and rearrangements of the TOP-I gene) [58–67] (table 1). In vitro data suggest that decreased activity of carboxylesterase may also alter the antitumor activity of irinotecan due to decreased enzymatical conversion of irinotecan to its active metabolite SN-38 [68]. Increased topoisomerase II expression has also been related to resistance to TOP-I interactive agents, data which are of interest because TOP-II has been shown to compensate for TOP-I function [60, 69, 70].

Furthermore, positively charged camptothecin derivatives (e.g., topotecan) may be transported by the MDR1 gene product P_{170}-glycoprotein and by the multidrug-resistance protein (MRP). However, in vivo both drug transporters appear not to confer significant resistance to irinotecan or SN-38 [71–75]. Decreased drug accumulation and resistance to camptothecins has also been observed recently in cell lines lacking MRP and P_{170}-glycoprotein expression [76–78]. In two of these topotecan- or mitoxantrone-selected cell lines (T8 and MX3, respectively) a new ATP-binding cassette (ABC) membrane transporter protein, termed BCRP/MXR/ABCP, was identified [78, 79].

Table 1. Cellular mechanisms of resistance to topoisomerase-I interactive agents

Cellular target	Mechanism of resistance
Topoisomerase-I	down-regulation of TOP-I gene, mRNA and protein point mutations, deletions and rearrangements of TOP-I gene altered structure and function of TOP-I phosphorylation state (e.g., role of protein kinase C)? interaction of nuclear proteins? induction of multi-ubiquitin TOP-I conjugates (e.g., 26S proteasome)?
Pgp-170 MRP BCRP/MXR/ABCP	decreased drug accumulation (e.g. topotecan)
Carboxylesterase activity	altered conversion of irinotecan to SN-38
UDP-glucuronosyltransferase	conjugation of SN-38 into its almost inactive glucuronide
Others	apoptosis (e.g., Bax/Bcl-2, c-myc, p53) cell cycle perturbations specific DNA repair

Pharmacokinetics of Irinotecan

Irinotecan undergoes extensive hepatic biotransformation with sequential metabolism: a) carboxylesterases convert irinotecan into its active metabolite SN-38; b) UDP-glucuronosyltransferase transforms SN-38 into its almost inactive glucuronide (7-ethyl-10-hydroxycamptothecin-glucuronide conjugate), and c) CYP3A metabolizes irinotecan into APC (7-ethyl-10-[4-N-(5-aminopentanoicacid)-1-piperidino] carbonyloxy-camptothecin) and NPC (7-ethyl-10-[4-N-(1-piperidino)-1-amino]-carbonyloxy-camptothecin) [80–85]. The plasma availabilities of these metabolites vary, with a plasma peak between 1 and 6 hours after i.v. short-time infusion [80–82].

Irinotecan undergoes renal and fecal elimination [82, 86]. The cumulative urine recovery of irinotecan and its metabolites ranged from 14 to 17% after 24 hours [82, 87]. The fecal excretion is about 30% within 56 hours, with most of the derivatives being excreted from 5 to 24 hours after administration [82]. As in plasma, irinotecan is the most predominant substance in urine and feces followed by APC and SN-38-G [86].

Independent of the schedule of drug administration diarrhea induced by irinotecan represents one of the most common dose-limiting toxicities. There is evidence that SN-38 glucuronide is hydrolyzed by intestinal ß-glucuronidase to active SN-38, which may damage intestinal epithelium cells [88, 89].

Cellular Interactions of Irinotecan with Other Drugs

In preclinical studies, schedule-dependent cytotoxic interactions have been reported for the combination of irinotecan with either thymidylate synthase (TS) inhibitors, platinum-derivatives or taxanes [90–100].

In vitro data showed a cytotoxic synergism for the sequence SN-38 followed by 5-FU, while the opposite sequence resulted in additive or antagonistic cytotoxic interactions [91, 93–95]. In cell culture, irinotecan itself produced synergistic cytotoxic interactions for the sequence irinotecan (IC_{20}) followed by 5-FU (IC_{50}) associated with increased DNA damage [93].

The antitumor activity of 5-FU in combination with irinotecan was also evaluated in several in vivo tumor models [96, 97], demonstrating that the schedule of irinotecan followed by 5-FU was the most active one. Similar results were observed in 5-FU (bolus) resistant colon tumor xenografts in nude mice, demonstrating increased therapeutic efficacy for the schedule irinotecan followed by 5-FU bolus [96]. The synergism of the sequence SN-38 followed by 5-FU may be explained by a prolonged inhibition of thymidylate synthase and increased incorporation of 5-FU derivatives (e.g., FdUTP) into DNA [92, 95].

Short-term exposure to SN-38 followed by raltitrexed, a specific and potent direct inhibitor of TS, may also result in cytotoxic synergism at broad dose-effect ranges in vitro, data which are similar to those obtained for 5-FU [90]. The opposite sequence of raltitrexed followed by SN-38 or a simultaneous exposure resulted in almost additive cytotoxic interactions.

The cellular pharmacology of the combination of SN-38 with the diaminocyclohexane platinum derivative oxaliplatin has been recently described [98, 99]. The combination of SN-38 and oxaliplatin showed in vitro cytotoxic synergism in the colon cancer cell line HT29, with a maximum effect when oxaliplatin was administered first [98]. The molecular mechanism of this synergism was explained by altered oxaliplatin interstrand cross-links repair machinery. In contrast, results obtained in HCT-8 colon tumor cells showed that the sequence of SN-38 followed by oxaliplatin was associated with synergistic cytotoxic interactions, while the opposite sequence resulted in antagonism [99].

The schedule docetaxel followed by SN-38 resulted in synergistic cytotoxic interactions in the non-small cell lung cancer cell line H460, associated with increased induction of protein-linked DNA breaks and decreased cytosolic accumulation of SN-38. In this model, no effects of docetaxel on TOP-I and -II expression were observed [100].

Conclusions

With the recognition that TOP-I is an important therapeutic target in cancer therapy, irinotecan is under an intensive clinical evaluation, primarily in patients with gastrointestinal cancer.

Based on promising preclinical data on synergistic cytotoxic drug interactions, a variety of irinotecan-based combinations are currently under clinical evaluation (e.g. cisplatin, oxaliplatin, raltitrexed, taxanes, capecitabine). However, further studies will have to address the question of the optimal use of these combinations. In addition, the task of future trials will be to identify molecular markers, which could be predictive for tumor response to irinotecan and irinotecan-based combinations.

Acknowledgements

Supported in part by a grant from Aventis Pharma, Bad Soden, Germany.

References

1 Chen AY, Liu LF: DNA topoisomerases: Essential enzymes and lethal targets. Annu Rev Pharmacol Toxicol 1994;34:191–218.
2 Lavelle F, Bissery MC, André S, et al: Preclinical evaluation of CPT-11 and its active metabolite SN-38. Semin Oncol 1996;23(suppl 3):11–20.
3 Pommier Y: Eukaryotic DNA topoisomerase I: Genome gatekeeper and its intruders, camptothecins. Semin Oncol 1996;23(suppl 3):3–10.
4 Wisemann LR, Markham A: Irinotecan: A review of its pharmacological properties and clinical efficacy in the management of advanced colorectal cancer. Drugs 1996;52:606–623.
5 Rothenberg ML: Topoisomerase I inhibitors: Review and update. Ann Oncol 1997;8:837–855.
6 Bleiberg H: CPT-11 in gastrointestinal cancer. Eur J Cancer 1999;35:371–379.
7 O'Leary J, Muggia FM: Camptothecins: A review of their development and schedules of administration. Eur J Cancer 1998;34:1500–1508.
8 Conti JA, Kemeny NE, Saltz LB, et al: Irinotecan is an active agent in untreated patients with metastatic colorectal cancer. J Clin Oncol 1996;14:709–715.
9 Pitot HC, Wender DB, O'Connell MJ, et al: Phase II trial of irinotecan in patients with metastatic colorectal carcinoma. J Clin Oncol 1997;8:2910–2919.
10 Pozzo C, Pyrhönen S, Bodrogi I, et al: A randomized phase II trial assessing irinotecan (IRI) and 5FU/folinic acid (LV), 'Mayo regimen', in first line palliative chemotherapy patients with metastatic colorectal cancer. Eur J Cancer 1999;35(suppl 4): S70(abstr).
11 Rougier P, Bugat R, Douillard JY, et al: Phase II study of irinotecan in the treatment of advanced colorectal cancer in chemotherapy-naïve patients and patients pretreated with fluorouracil-based chemotherapy. J Clin Oncol 1997;15:251–260.
12 Van Cutsem E, Rougier P, Droz JP, et al: Clinical benefit of irinotecan (CPT-11) in metastatic colorectal cancer resistant to 5-FU. Proc Am Soc Clin Oncol 1997;16:268a (abstr).
13 Von Hoff DD; Rothenberg ML, Pitot HC, et al: Irinotecan (CPT-11) therapy for patients with previously treated metastatic colorectal cancer: Overall results of FDA-reviewed pivotal US clinical trials. Proc Am Soc Clin Oncol 1997;16:228a (abstr).
14 Conroy T: Single-agent chemotherapy of colorectal cancer; in Bleiberg H, Rougier P, Wilke H (eds): Management of Colorectal Cancer. London, Dunitz, 1998, pp 211–220.
15 Saltz LB, Locker PK, Pirotta N, et al: Weekly irinotecan (CPT-11), leucovorin (LV), and fluorouracil (FU) is superior to daily x5 LV/FU in patients with previously untreated metastatic colorectal cancer. Proc Am Soc Clin Oncol 1999;18:233a (abstr).
16 Pommier Y, Pourquier P, Fan Y, et al: Mechanism of action of eukaryotic DNA topoisomerase I and drugs targeted to the enzyme. Biochim Biophys Acta 1998:1400:83–106.
17 Wang JC: DNA topoisomerases. Annu Rev Biochem 1996;65:635–692.
18 Redinbo MR, Stewart L, Kuhn P, et al: Crystal structures of human topoisomerase I in covalent and noncovalent complexes with DNA. Science 1998:279:1504–1513.
19 Stewart L, Redinbo MR, Qiu X, et al: A model for the mechanism of human topoisomerase I. Science 1998; 279:1534–1541.
20 Takahashi M, Matsuda M, Kojima A, et al: Human immunodeficiency virus type 1 reverse transcriptase: Enhancement of activity by interaction with cellular topoisomerase I. Proc Natl Acad Sci USA 1995;92:5694–5698.
21 Heiland S, Knippers R, Kunze N: The promoter region of the human type-I-DNA-topoisomerase gene. Protein-binding sites and sequences involved in transcriptional regulation. Eur J Biochem 1993; 217:813–822.
22 Kunze N, Klein M, Richter A, et al: Structural characterization of the human DNA topoisomerase I gene promoter. Eur J Biochem 1990;194: 323–330.
23 Kunze N, Yang G, Dölberg M, et al: Structure of the human type I DNA topoisomerase gene. J Biol Chem 1991;266:9610–9616.
24 Romig H, Richter A: Expression of the type I DNA topoisomerase gene in adenovirus-5 infected human cells. Nucleic Acids Res 1990;18:801–808.
25 Rosenberg BH, Ungers G, Deutsch JF: Variation in DNA swivel enzyme activity during the mammalian cell cycle. Nucleic Acids Res 1976;12:3305–3311.
26 Sobczak J, Tournier MF, Lotti AM, et al: Gene expression in regenerating liver in relation to cell proliferation and stress. Eur J Biochem 1989;180: 49–53.
27 Heiland S, Knippers R: The human topoisomerase I gene promoter is regulated by NF-IL6. Mol Cell Biol 1995;12:6623–6631.
28 Leteurtre F, Kohlhagen G, Fesen MR, et al: Effects of DNA methylation on topoisomerase I and II cleavage activities. J Biol Chem 1994;269:7893–7900.
29 Piret B, Schoonbroodt S, Piette J: The ATM protein is required for sustained activation of NF-kappaB following DNA damage. Oncogene 1999;13: 2261–2271.
30 Pommier Y, Kerrigan D, Hartman KD, et al: Phosphorylation of mammalian DNA topoisomerase I and activation by protein kinase C. J Biol Chem 1990;16:9418–9422.
31 Samuels DS, Shimizu Y, Shimizu N: Protein kinase C phosphorylates DNA topoisomerase I. FEBS Lett 1989;259:57–60.
32 Durban E, Goodenough M, Mills J: Topoisomerase I phosphorylation in vitro and in rapidly growing Novihoff hepatoma cells. EMBO J 1985;4:2921–2926.
33 Rivory LP, Bowles MR, Robert J, et al: Conversion of irinotecan (CPT-11) to its active metabolite, 7-ethyl-10-hydroxy-camptothecin (SN-38), by human liver carboxylesterase. Biochem Pharmacol 1996; 52:1103–1111.
34 Satoh R, Hosokawa M, Atsumi R, et al: Metabolic activation of CPT-11, 7-ethyl-10-[4-(1-piperidino)-1-piperidino]carbonyloxycamptothecin, a novel antitumor agent, by carboxylesterase. Biol Pharm Bull 1994;17:662–664.
35 Covey JM, Jaxel C, Kohn KW, et al: Protein-linked DNA strand breaks induced in mammalian cells by camptothecin, an inhibitor of topoisomerase I. Cancer Res 1989;49:5016–5022.
36 Fan Y, Weinstein JN, Kohn KW, et al: Molecular modeling studies of the DNA- topoisomerase I ternary cleavable complex with camptothecin. J Med Chem 1998;41:2216–2226.
37 Hsiang YH, Liu LF: Identification of mammalian DNA topoisomerase I as an intracellular target of the anticancer drug camptothecin. Cancer Res 1988;48:1722–1726.
38 Hsiang YH, Lihou MG, Liu LF: Arrest of replication forks by drug-stabilized topoisomerase I-DNA cleavable complexes as a mechanism of cell killing by camptothecin. Cancer Res 1989;49:5077–5082.
39 Ryan AJ, Squires S, Strutt HL, et al: Different fates of camptothecin-induced replication fork-associated double-strand DNA breaks in mammalian cells. Carcinogenesis 1994;15:823–828.

40 Tsao YP, Russo A, Nyamuswa G, et al: Interaction between replication forks and topoisomerase I-DNA cleavable complexes: Studies in a cell-free SV40 DNA replication system. Cancer Res 1993; 53:5908–5914.

41 Ryan AJ, Squires S, Strutt HL, et al: Camptothecin cytotoxicity in mammalian cells is associated with the induction of persistent double strand breaks in replicating DNA. Nucleic Acids Res 1991;19:3295–3300.

42 Egyházi E, Durban E: Microinjection of anti-topoisomerase I immunglobulin G into nuclei of Chironomus tentans salivary gland cells leads to blockage of transcription elongation. Mol Cell Biol 1987; 7:4308–4316.

43 Zhang H, Wang JC, Liu LF: Involvement of DNA topoisomerase I in transcription of human ribosomal RNA genes. Proc Natl Acad Sci USA 1988;85: 1060–1064.

44 Houghton PJ, Cheshire PJ, Hallman JD, et al: Efficacy of topoisomerase I inhibitors, topotecan and irinotecan, administered at low dose levels in protracted schedules to mice bearing xenografts of human tumors. Cancer Chemother Pharmacol 1995; 36:393–403.

45 Houghton PJ, Cheshire PJ, Hallman JC, et al: Therapeutic efficacy of the topoisomerase I inhibitor 7-ethyl-10-(4-[1-piperidino]-1-piperidino]-carbonyloxy-camptothecin against human tumor xenografts: Lack of cross-resistance in vivo in tumors with acquired resistance to the topoisomerase I inhibitor 9-dimethylaminomethyl-10-hydroxycamptothecin. Cancer Res 1993;53: 2823–2829.

46 Jansen WJ, Zwart B, Hulscher ST, et al: CPT-11 in human colon-cancer cell lines and xenografts: Characterization of cellular sensitivity determinants. Int J Cancer 1997;70:335–340.

47 McLeod HL, Keith WN: Variation in topoisomerase I gene copy number as a mechanism for intrinsic drug sensitivity. Br J Cancer 1996;74:508–512.

48 Pommier Y, Leteurtre F, Fesen MR, et al: Cellular determinants of sensitivity and resistance to DNA topoisomerase inhibitors. Cancer Invest 1994;12: 530–542.

49 Giovanella BC, Stehlin JS, Wall ME, et al: DNA topoisomerase I-targeted chemotherapy of human cancer in xenografts. Science 1989;246:1046–1048.

50 Husain I, Mohler JL, Seigerl HF, et al: Elevation of topoisomerase I mRNA, protein, and catalytic activity in human tumors: Demonstration of tumor-type specificity and implications for cancer chemotherapy. Cancer Res 1994;54:539–546.

51 Staley BE, Samowitz WS, Bronstein IB, et al: Expression of DNA topoisomerase I and DNA topoisomerase II-alpha in carcinoma of the colon. Mod Pathol 1999;12:356–361.

52 Takatani H, Oka M, Fukuda M, et al: Gene mutation analysis and quantitation of DNA topoisomerase I in previously untreated non-small cell lung carcinomas. Jpn J Cancer Res 1997;88:160–165.

53 van der Zee AGJ, Hollema H, de Jong S, et al: P-glycoprotein expression and DNA topoisomerase I and II activity in benign tumors of the ovary and in malignant tumors of the ovary, before and after platinum/cyclophosphamide chemotherapy. Cancer Res 1991;51:5915–5920.

54 McLeod HL, Douglas F, Oates M, et al: Topoisomerase I and II activity in human breast, cervix, lung and colon cancer. Int J Cancer 1994;59:607–611.

55 Goldwasser F, Bae I, Valenti M, et al: Topoisomerase I-related parameters and camptothecin activity in the colon carcinoma cell lines from the National Cancer Institute anticancer screen. Cancer Res 1995;55:2116–2121.

56 Chen SF, Rothenberg ML, Clark G, et al: Human tumor carboxylesterase activity correlates with CPT-11 cytotoxicity in vitro. Proc Am Assoc Cancer Res 1994;35:365 (abstr).

57 Ohashi N, Fujiwara Y, Yamaoka N, et al: No alteration in DNA topoisomerase I gene related to CPT-11 resistance in human lung cancer. Jpn J Cancer Res 1996;87:1280–1287.

58 Andoh T, Ishii K, Suzuki Y, et al: Characterization of a mammalian mutant with a camptothecin-resistant DNA topoisomerase I. Proc Natl Acad Sci 1987;84:5565–5569.

59 Benedetti P, Fiorani P, Capuani L, et al: Camptothecin resistance from a single mutation changing glycine 363 of human DNA topoisomerase I to cysteine. Cancer Res 1993;53:4343–4348.

60 Eng WK, McCabe FL, Tan KB, et al: Development of a stable camptothecin-resistant subline of P388 leukemia with reduced topoisomerase I content. Mol Pharmacol 1990;38:471–480.

61 Fujimori A, Harker WG, Kohlhagen G, et al: Mutation at the catalytic site of topoisomerase I in CEM/C2, a human leukemia cell line resistant to camptothecin. Cancer Res 1995;55:1339–1346.

62 Gromova II, Kjeldsen E, Svejstrup JQ, et al: Characterization of an altered DNA catalysis of a camptothecin-resistant eukaryotic topoisomerase I. Nucleic Acids Res 1993;21:593–600.

63 Kanzawa F, Sugimoto Y, Minato K, et al: Establishment of a camptothecin analogue (CPT-11)-resistant cell line of human non-small cell lung cancer: Characterization and mechanism of resistance. Cancer Res 1990;50:5919–5924.

64 Kapoor R, Slade DL, Fujimori A, et al: Altered topoisomerase I expression in two subclones of human CEM leukemia selected for resistance to camptothecin. Oncol Res 1995;7:83–95.

65 Sorenson M, Sehested M, Jensen PB: Characterisation of a human small-cell lung cancer cell line resistant to the DNA topoisomerase I-directed drug topotecan. Br J Cancer 1995;72:399–404.

66 Sugimoto Y, Tsukahara S, Oh-hara T, et al: Decreased expression of DNA topoisomerase I in camptothecin-resistant tumor cell lines as determined by a monoclonal antibody. Cancer Res 1990; 50:6925–6930.

67 Tan KB, Mattern MR, Eng WK, et al: Nonproductive rearrangement of DNA topoisomerase I and II genes: Correlation with resistance to topoisomerase inhibitors. J Natl Cancer Inst 1989;81:1732–1735.

68 Kojima A, Hackett NR, Crystal RG: Reversal of CPT-11 resistance of lung cancer cells by adenovirus-mediated gene transfer of the human carboxylesterase cDNA. Cancer Res 1998;58:4368–4374.

69 Friedman HS, Dolan ME, Kaufmann SH, et al: Elevated DNA polymerase alpha, DNA polymerase beta, and DNA topoisomerase II in a melphalan-resistant rhabdomyosarcoma xenograft that is cross-resistant to nitrosoureas and topotecan. Cancer Res 1994;54:3487–3493.

70 Sugimoto Y, Tsukahara S, Oh-hara T, et al: Elevated expression of DNA topoisomerase II in camptothecin-resistant human tumor cell lines. Cancer Res 1990;50:7962–7965.

71 Hendricks CB, Rowinsky EK, Grochow LB, et al: Effect of P-glycoprotein expression on the accumulation and cytotoxicity of topotecan (SK and F104864), a new camptothecin analogue. Cancer Res 1992;52:2268–2278.

72 Jansen WJM, Hulscher TM, van Ark-Otte J, et al: CPT-11 sensitivity in relation to the expression of P170-glycoprotein and multidrug resistance-associated protein. Br J Cancer 1998;77:359–365.

73 Hapke G, Vanhoefer U, Harstrick A, et al: Antitumor efficacy of irinotecan (CPT-11) and topotecan in nude mice bearing tumor xenografts that express the multidrug resistance protein (MRP). Onkologie 1999;22(suppl 1):219 (abstr).

74 Vanhoefer U, Müller MR, Hilger RA, et al: Reversal of MDR1-associated resistance to topotecan by PAK-200S, a new dihydropyridine analogue, in human cancer cell lines. Br J Cancer 1999;81:1304–1310.

75 Mattern MR, Hofmann GA, Polsky RM, et al: In vitro and in vivo effects of clinically important camptothecin analogues on multidrug-resistant cells. Oncol Res 1993;5:467–474.

76 Ma J, Maliepaard M, Nooter K, et al: Reduced cellular accumulation of topotecan: A novel mechanism of resistance in a human ovarian cancer cell line. Br J Cancer 1998;77:1645–1652.

77 Yang CHJ, Horton JK, Cowan KH, et al: Cross-resistance to camptothecin analogues in a mitoxantrone-resistant human breast carcinoma cell line is not due to DNA topoisomerase I alterations. Cancer Res 1995;55:4004–4009.

78 Maliepaard M, van Gastelen MA, de Jong LA, et al: Overexpression of the BCRP/MXR/ABCP gene in a topotecan-selected ovarian tumor cell line. Cancer Res 1999;59:4559–4563.

79 Brangi M, Litman T, Ciotti M, et al: Camptothecin resistance: Role of the ATP-binding cassette (ABC), mitoxantrone-resistance half-transporter (MXR), and potential for glucuronidation in MXR-expressing cells. Cancer Res 1999;59:5938–5946.

80 Gupta E, Mick R, Ramirez J, et al: Pharmacokinetic and pharmacodynamic evaluation of the topoisomerase inhibitor irinotecan in cancer patients. J Clin Oncol 1997;15:1502–1510.

81 Rivory LP, Haaz MC, Canal P, et al: Pharmacokinetic interrelationships of irinotecan (CPT-11) and its three major plasma metabolites in patients enrolled in phase I/II trials. Clin Cancer Res 1997;3: 1261–1266.

82 Sparreboom A, de Jonge MJA, de Bruijn P, et al: Irinotecan (CPT-11) metabolism and disposition in cancer patients. Clin Cancer Res 1998;4:2747–2754.

83 Canal P, Gay C, Dezeuze A, et al: Pharmacokinetics and pharmacodynamics of irinotecan during a phase II clinical trial in colorectal cancer. J Clin Oncol 1996;4:2688–2695.

84 Haaz MC, Dodds HM, Riou JF, et al: Identification of a new metabolite of CPT-11 (irinotecan). Biosynthesis and activation to SN-38 by human hepatic microsomes. Ann Oncol 1998;9(suppl 2):58 (abstr).

85 Raymond E, Vernillet L, Boige V, et al: Phase I and pharmacokinetic study of irinotecan (CPT-11) in cancer patients with hepatic dysfunction. Proc Am Soc Clin Oncol 1999;18:634 (abstr).

86 Schaaf L, Slatter JG, Sams J, et al: Metabolism and excretion of irinotecan (CPT-11) following IV infusion of [^{14}C]CPT-11 in patients with advanced solid tumor malignancy. Proc Am Soc Clin Oncol 1999;18:164a (abstr).

87 Chabot GG, Abigerges D, Catimel G, et al: Population pharmacokinetics and pharmacodynamics of irinotecan (CPT-11) and active metabolite SN-38 during phase I trials. Ann Oncol 1995;6:141–151.
88 Takasuna K, Hagiwara T, Hirohashi M, et al: Involvement of ß-glucuronidase in intestinal microflora in the intestinal toxicity of the antitumor camptothecin derivative irinotecan hydrochloride (CPT-11) in rats. Cancer Res 1996;56:3752–3757.
89 Takasuna K, Hagiwara T, Hirohashi M, et al: Inhibition of intestinal microflora ß-glucuronidase modifies the distribution of the active metabolite of the antitumor agent, irinotecan hydrochloride (CPT-11) in rats. Cancer Chemother Pharmacol 1998;42:280–286.
90 Aschele C, Baldo C, Sobrero AF, et al: Schedule-dependent synergism between raltitrexed and irinotecan in human colon cancer cells in vitro. Clin Cancer Res 1998;4:1323–1330.
91 Guichard S, Cussac D, Hennebelle I, et al: Sequence-dependent activity of the irinotecan-5FU combination in human colon-cancer model HT-29 in vitro and in vivo. Int J Cancer 1997;73:729–734.
92 Guichard S, Hennebelle I, Bugat R, et al: Cellular interactions of 5-fluorouracil and the camptothecin analogue CPT-11 (irinotecan) in a human colorectal carcinoma cell line. Biochem Pharmacol 1998;55:667–676.
93 Mans DRA, Grivicich I, Peters GJ, et al: Sequence-dependent growth inhibition and DNA damage formation by the irinotecan-5-fluorouracil combination in human colon carcinoma cell lines. Eur J Cancer 1999;35:1851–1861.
94 Mullany S, Svingen PA, Kaufmann SH, et al: Effect of adding the topoisomerase I poison 7-ethyl-10-hydroxycamptothecin (SN38) to 5-fluorouracil and folinic acid in HCT-8 cells: Elevated dTTP pools and enhanced cytotoxicity. Cancer Chemother Pharmacol 1999;42:391–399.
95 Pavillard V, Formento P, Rostagno P, et al: Combination of irinotecan (CPT-11) and 5-fluorouracil with an analysis of cellular determinants of drug activity. Biochem Pharmacol 1998;56:1315–1322.
96 Vanhoefer U, Hapke G, Harstrick A, et al: Schedule-dependent antitumor efficacy of irinotecan (CPT-11) in 5-FU resistant human colon tumor xenograft HT29R1. Proc Am Assoc Cancer Res 1999;40:110 (abstr).
97 Rustum YM, Cao S: New drugs in therapy of colorectal cancer: Preclinical studies. Semin Oncol 1999;26:612–620.
98 Zeghari-Squalli N, Raymond E, Cvitkovic E, et al: Cellular pharmacology of the combination of the DNA topoisomerase I inhibitor SN-38 and the diaminocyclohexane platinum derivative oxaliplatin. Clin Cancer Res 1999;5:1189–1196.
99 Erlichman C, Boerner S, Kaufmann SH: Mechanism of synergy between oxaliplatin and the topoisomerase I inhibitor SN-38. Clin Cancer Res 1999: 5(suppl):3853 (abstr).
100 Vanhoefer U, Hilger RA, Harstrick A, et al: Schedule-dependent cytotoxic interactions of irinotecan (SN-38) and docetaxel in human non-small-cell lung cancer (NSCLC). Clin Cancer Res 1999:5(suppl):3859–3860 (abstr).

ONKOLOGIE

Onkologie 2000;23(suppl 4):8–14

Irinotecan: New Results in the Combination Chemotherapy of Colorectal Cancer

H. Wilke[a] U. Vanhoefer[b] W. Achterrath[c] M. Stahl[a]

[a]Klinik für Innere Medizin und Internistische Onkologie/Hämatologie, Kliniken Essen-Mitte
[b]Innere Klinik (Tumorforschung), Universitätsklinik Essen
[c]Aventis, Department of Clinical Research, Oncology-New Technology, Bad Soden

Key Words
Irinotecan · Combination chemotherapy · Colorectal cancer

Summary
Irinotecan is one of the newer cytostatic agents which have a clinically relevant antineoplastic activity in colorectal cancer. As single-agent irinotecan induced an overall objective response rate of about 25% in chemonaive patients and of about 13% in 5-fluorouracil (5-FU)-pretreated patients.
In the past years an increasing number of various combinations of irinotecan with oxaliplatin, tomudex and especially 5-FU/folinic acid (FA) were investigated in phase I/II/III trials. These trials showed that these combinations are active and that the toxicity profile is acceptable and manageable. In phase II trials combinations of irinotecan plus 5-FU/FA induced overall objective response rates of 40–70% in chemonaive patients and of 20–30% in patients with prior 5-FU-based chemotherapies. Two large randomized trials compared the combination of irinotecan plus either bolus 5-FU/FA or 'infusional' 5-FU/FA with 5-FU/FA alone as first-line chemotherapy for metastatic disease. These two trials consistently showed that the combination was statistically significantly superior to 5-FU/FA alone concerning the induction of objective responses (39 vs. 21% and 35 vs. 21%), median time to progression (7.0 vs. 4.3 months and 6.7 vs. 4.4 months), and median survival (14.8 vs. 12.6 months and 17.4 vs. 14.1 months). Quality of life analysis performed in both studies did not show that adding irinotecan to 5-FU/FA had a negative impact on overall quality of life parameters of the patients. Based on these study results, the combination of irinotecan plus 5-FU/FA has to be considered as a new standard first-line treatment for patients with metastatic colorectal cancer.

Schlüsselwörter
Irinotecan · Kombinationschemotherapie · Kolorektales Karzinom

Zusammenfassung
Irinotecan ist eines der neueren Zytostatika, die beim kolorektalen Karzinom eine klinisch relevante neoplastische Wirksamkeit aufweisen. Als Monosubstanz induzierte Irinotecan bei unvorbehandelten und bei vorbehandelten Patienten eine objektive Remissionsrate von 25 bzw. 13%.
Mittlerweile sind eine Vielzahl unterschiedlicher Kombinationen von Irinotecan mit Oxaliplatin, Tomudex und speziell mit 5-Fluorouracil (5-FU)/Folinsäure (FA) in Phase-I/II/III-Studien geprüft worden. Hierbei zeigte sich nicht nur, dass diese Kombinationen gut wirksam sind, sondern auch, dass sie ein akzeptables Nebenwirkungsprofil aufweisen. Mit Kombinationen von Irinotecan/5-FU/FA wurden in Phase-II-Studien bei unvorbehandelten Patienten objektive Remissionsraten von 40–70% und bei 5-FU-vorbehandelten Patienten von 20–30% induziert. In zwei großen randomisierten Studien, in denen eine Kombination aus Bolus-5-FU/FA oder «infusional» 5-FU/FA plus Irinotecan mit 5-FU/FA allein verglichen wurde, erwies sich die Kombinationschemotherapie der alleinigen 5-FU/FA-Therapie als statistisch signifikant überlegen, bezogen auf die Rate an objektiven Remissionen (39 vs. 21% und 35 vs. 21%), auf die mediane Zeit bis zur Tumorprogression (7,0 versus 4,3 Monate und 6,7 versus 4,4 Monate) und auf die mediane Überlebenszeit (14,8 versus 12,6 Monate und 17,4 vs. 14,1 Monate). Die in diesen Studien durchgeführten Lebensqualitätsanalysen zeigten, dass das Hinzufügen von Irinotecan zu 5-FU/FA keinen negativen Einfluss auf die Lebensqualität der Patienten hatte. Aufgrund dieser Studien ist die Kombination Irinotecan/5-FU/FA als die neue Standard-First-line-Therapie des kolorektalen Karzinoms anzusehen.

KARGER

Fax +49 761 4 52 07 14
E-mail Information@Karger.de
www.karger.com

Accessible online at:
www.karger.com/journals/onk

Prof. Hansjochen Wilke
Klinik für Innere Medizin I und Internistische Onkologie/Hämatologie
Kliniken Essen-Mitte
Henricistraße 92
D-45136 Essen (Germany)

Introduction

During the past decades the overall prognosis of colorectal cancer (CRC) has not essentially changed. CRC remains one of the major causes of cancer death in developed countries, and about 40–50% of CRC patients will die of their disease, predominantly due to metastatic spread. Until the late 1980s, therapeutic options for patients with advanced colorectal cancer have almost exclusively been based on fluoropyrimidines. Single-agent 5-fluorouracil (5-FU), predominantly administered as i.v. bolus injection, was the standard of care for more than 30 years and was replaced since the early 1990s by the combination of 5-FU plus folinic acid (FA), which demonstrated a higher antineoplastic activity than 5-FU alone [1]. With bolus 5-FU/FA, which was either administered five times daily every 4 weeks (Mayo regimen) or once weekly ×6 (Roswell Park regimen), an overall response rate of about 20% and median survival times of 12 months were achieved [1]. Further improvements in the systemic treatment of CRC occurred with the introduction of infusional 5-FU/FA regimens administered once weekly as a 24- or 48-hour infusion or as a biweekly 48-hour infusional schedule. Compared with bolus 5-FU/FA, infusional 5-FU/FA induced higher response rates (30–40%), longer progression-free intervals/times to progression (6–7 months), and median survival times up to 17 months [2, 3]. In the past decade a number of new compounds, such as oxaliplatin, tomudex, oral 5-FU prodrugs (capecitabine, UFT, S1) and irinotecan, which demonstrated activity in CRC have been developed and introduced into the clinic.

Irinotecan: Clinical Activity

Irinotecan (CPT-11) is a semisynthetic derivative of the natural alkaloid camptothecin and belongs to a new class of antineoplastic agents, called topoisomerase-I interactive compounds [4–7]. Since its introduction into the clinic, irinotecan has undergone a comprehensive evaluation as single agent, and in combination chemotherapy in first-line as well as in second-line therapy of CRC.
Irinotecan was evaluated as first-line chemotherapy in Europe and in the US in four nonrandomized phase II studies with a total of 175 response-evaluable patients [8–11]. A mean overall response rate of 24% has been achieved with the 'European' once-every-three-weeks schedule and of 29% with the 'US' weekly-times-four schedule. The median response duration ranged from 8 to 9 months, and the median survival time was 12 months. Randomized trials comparing irinotecan with bolus 5-FU/FA showed that irinotecan was at least equally effective as the generally accepted standard bolus 5-FU/FA [12, 13].
Clinically relevant activity was also shown in patients who had failed to respond to prior 5-FU/FA therapy. With the abovementioned irinotecan schedules an overall response rate of 13% (95% [confidence interval] CI 11–15%) and a tumor growth control rate (CR/PR/NC) of 50% (95% CI 47–53%) were achieved in more than 1,300 patients treated in 15 studies [9, 10, 14–25]. Median response duration ranged from 6 to 8 months and median survival times from 7 to 13 months. The clinical benefit of second-line irinotecan as assumed from these data was confirmed by two randomized trials which compared irinotecan either with best supportive care or with the best estimated infusional 5-FU regimen in patients with resistance to conventional 5-FU regimens [26, 27]. The encouraging single-agent activity of irinotecan led to broad investigation of irinotecan-containing combinations in CRC.

Irinotecan in Combination with Other Cytotoxic Drugs

Phase I Trials

Irinotecan in combination with fluoropyrimidines +/– FA: In association with bolus 5-FU +/– FA, irinotecan was investigated in four different dose and time schedules [28–40]. The recommended doses that were determined in the various phase I trials are listed in table 1. The dose-limiting toxicities of these bolus 5-FU/FA + irinotecan regimens were either neutropenia or a combination of neutropenia and diarrhea.
These phase I studies suggested that irinotecan can be combined with various 5-FU regimens and prompted the initiation of further phase I studies using irinotecan in combination with higher doses of 5-FU +/– FA, given as i.v. infusion over 24 or 48 h [28, 38, 39] (table 1). When all drugs were administered in a weekly-times-six schedule, the dose-limiting toxicity was diarrhea for the 24-hour application of 5-FU/FA [39] and was not yet reached for the 48-hour schedule [28]. With a biweekly schedule of irinotecan plus 5-FU/FA (De Gramont schedule), the dose-limiting toxicities were neutropenia and diarrhea [31], and with a once-every-three-weeks schedule of irinotecan in combination with leucovorin-modulated 5-FU over 48 h the dose-limiting toxicity again consisted of a combination of neutropenia and diarrhea [32]. In these trials with irinotecan and infusional 5-FU/FA significant response rates were observed. Overall responses of 69% have been achieved in first-line treatment of CRC with the combination using irinotecan and infusional 5-FU/FA given as the once-weekly-times-six 24-hour schedule [39]. In patients with 5-FU-pretreated colon cancer, response rates of 23 and 33% have been reported for irinotecan in combination with 5-FU/FA (De-Gramont schedule) or with irinotecan plus chronomodulated 5-FU/FA, respectively [31, 34].
Table 2 summarizes results of phase I trials combining irinotecan with 5-FU given as continuous infusion over several days with or without FA [34, 35, 37].
Irinotecan was combined with tomudex in two phase I studies in patients with solid tumors [41, 42]. Asthenia was found as dose-limiting toxicity in both studies. The recommended doses

Table 1. Phase I studies of irinotecan (CPT-11) with 5-FU +/– FA

Ref.	Patients evaluable, n	Agent	Recommended doses, mg/m^2	Schedule	Dose-limiting toxicity
Irinotecan and 5-FU short-time infusion					
36	27	CPT-11	125 i.v.	weekly for 4 weeks	neutropenia
		FA	20 i.v.	weekly for 4 weeks	
		5-FU	500 i.v. bolus	for 4 weeks, q6 weeks	
30	31	CPT-11	200 i.v.	d1	neutropenia
		FA	250 i.v.	d2	diarrhea
		5-FU	850 i.v. bolus	d2; q2 weeks	
29	36	CPT-11	300 i.v.	d1	neutropenia
		5-FU	375 i.v. bolus	d1-5; q4 weeks	
33	47	CPT-11	275 i.v.	d1	neutropenia
		FA	20 i.v.	d2–5	diarrhea
		5-FU	400 i.v. 90 min	d2–5; q4 weeks	
Irinotecan with 5-FU 24 or 48 hours infusion					
38, 39	47	CPT-11	80 i.v.	weekly for 6 weeks	diarrhea
		FA	500 i.v.	weekly for 6 weeks	
		5-FU	2600 i.v. 24h	weekly for 6 weeks; q8 weeks	
31	55	CPT-11	180–200 i.v.	d1	not reached
		FA	200 i.v.	d1+2	
		5-FU	400 i.v.	bolus d1+2	
		5-FU	600 i.v.	22h d1+2; q2 weeks	
40	83	CPT-11	400 i.v.	d1	neutropenia
		FA	250 i.v.	d1	diarrhea
		5-FU	3500 i.v.	48h d1; q 3 weeks	
Irinotecan and 5-FU protracted infusion					
35	42	CPT-11	350 i.v.	d1	diarrhea
		5-FU	600 per day	d2–5 protracted infusion	neutropenia
34	26	CPT-11	350 i.v.	d1	neutropenia
		FA 150	per day as protracted infusion	over 5 days	diarrhea
		5-FU	700 /d as protracted infusion	for 5 days	
37	31	CPT-11	300 i.v.	d1	neutropenia
		5-FU	250 i.v. per day protracted infusion f	or 14 days	

Table 2. Randomized phase III trials with irinotecan, 5-FU and FA

Author	Study	Patients, n	cRR, %	p	mTTP, months	p	mS months	p
Douillard et al. (2000)	CPT-11/5-FU/FA	198	35	0.005	6.7	0.001	17.4	0.032
	5-FU/FA	187	21		4.4		14.1	
Saltz et al. (1999) + updated results (2000)	CPT-11/5-FU/FA	225	39	0.0001	7.0	0.004	14.8	0.042
	FU/FA	219	21		4.3		12.6	

cRR = Confirmed response rate; mTTP = median time to progression; mS = median survival.

were as follows: irinotecan 350 mg/m^2 and tomudex 3 mg/m^2 given once every three weeks.

Four phase I studies were performed with the combination of irinotecan and oxaliplatin in patients with advanced gastrointestinal tumors [43–45]. A once-every-two-weeks schedule and a once-every-three-weeks schedule were investigated in two separate studies each. Dose-limiting toxicity consisted of neutropenia for the 3-weekly schedule (recommended dose: irinotecan 200 mg/m^2, oxaliplatin 85 mg/m^2) and of neutropenia and diarrhea for the biweekly schedule (recommended dose: irinotecan 85 mg/m^2, oxaliplatin 175 mg/m^2). These combinations induced overall response rates of 29 and 55% in patients with colorectal cancer and prior exposure to 5-FU [43, 45].

Phase II Trials

Two phase II trials with irinotecan either 350 mg/m^2, day 1, q3 weeks or 100mg/m^2 weekly for 4 weeks alternated with the Mayo regime of 5-FU/FA were conducted as first-line chemotherapy in patients with advanced CRC [46, 47]. In both trials the overall response rate was about 30% and the median survival times were 16–18 months. Two other trials investigated irinotecan in combination with infusional 5-FU/FA. An overall response rate of 26% was achieved with irinotecan plus 5-FU/FA according to the De Gramont schedule [48] and a confirmed response rate of 72% was reported with a weekly-times-six schedule of irinotecan (80 mg/m^2) and a 24-hour infusion of 5-FU (2.0 g/m^2) + FA (200 mg/m^2) [49].

Two randomized trials compared irinotecan/5-FU/FA-based regimens with either 5-FU/FA administered according to the De Gramont or to the Mayo Clinic regimen as first-line chemotherapy for advanced disease [50, 51]. In one trial 102 patients received either the De Gramont regimen alone or the same 5-FU/FA schedule in combination with irinotecan. Responses were observed in 20 and 42% of evaluable patients, respectively [51]. The second study enrolled 117 patients and compared a weekly-times-four schedule of irinotecan at a dose of 125 mg/m^2 in combination with FA (20 mg/m^2)/5-FU (500 mg/m^2) (Saltz regimen) with either 350 mg/m^2 of irinotecan alternating with 5-FU/FA (Mayo regimen), or the Mayo regimen alone. The overall response rates were 47, 39 and 24%, respectively [50].

As salvage chemotherapy, the combination of irinotecan plus infusional 5-FU/FA (modified or original De Gramont schedule) was investigated in two nonrandomized phase II trials in patients with prior exposure to 5-FU/FA-based chemotherapies [52, 53]. Depending on the previous chemotherapy regimens, a response rate of 6% was achieved in patients who had failed to 5-FU/FA and 5-FU/FA/oxaliplatin (third-line chemotherapy) and a response rate of 22% was found in less extensively pretreated patients.

The combination of irinotecan plus oxaliplatin administered with G-CSF support induced an encouraging objective response rate of 42% in a phase II trial [54].

In a randomized phase II trial mitomycin was either combined with irinotecan or with oxaliplatin in a total of 64 response-evaluable patients failing 5-FU-based therapy [55]. The observed responses rates were similar with both regimens (21 and 16%). The median time to disease progression appeared to be longer with irinotecan/mitomycin (7.0 vs. 5.2 months).

Phase III Trials

The promising results being achieved with 5-FU/FA/irinotecan combinations in the phase I and II evaluation program prompted the initiation of two large randomized international trials comparing the efficacy, toxicity, and quality of life for this combination with more frequently used 5-FU/FA regimens alone as first-line chemotherapy in patients with metastatic CRC (table 2) [13, 56].

In the first trial which was conducted in the USA, Canada, Australia, and New Zealand a weekly combination of irinotecan, FA and 5-FU was chosen, based on the phase I trial reported by Saltz and coworkers [13, updated results]. The control arm with which this combination was compared was a conventional 5-FU/low-dose FA schedule (Mayo Clinic regimen). A third arm consisted of single-agent irinotecan. Due to the statistical design of this study a statistical comparison with the other two study arms was not planned for the irinotecan alone arm. Stratification criteria were performance status, age, time from diagnosis, and prior adjuvant therapy (> 12 months since completion of adjuvant 5-FU therapy). The statistical analysis involved time to progression (TTP) as the main end-point of the trial as well as time to treatment failure (TTF), response rate, overall survival, safety, and quality of life as secondary study end-points. The number of patients necessary for the statistical evaluation (220 patients per treatment arm) was based on the assumption that the 5-FU/FA/irinotecan treatment arm would be associated with a 40% improvement in TTP relative to the 5-FU/FA control arm. While the schedules of 5-FU administration were different, the trial was designed with the knowledge that the 5-FU dose intensity in the combination arm (333 mg/m^2/week) would be lower than the planned 531 mg/m^2/week in the control arm. This design helped to ensure that any incremental beneficial effects of the irinotecan/5-FU/FA regimen could be attributed definitively to irinotecan. From May 1996 until May 1998, a total of 683 patients were enrolled with similar numbers of patients in each treatment group. These patients constituted the intent-to-treat population on which all efficacy analysis were performed. Accounting for patients who were never treated or were treated on another treatment arm, the remaining 667 patients were analyzed for drug administration, safety, and quality of life. The treatment arms were well balanced for gender, median age, median performance status, and prior adjuvant therapy as well as for disease-related risk factors. Of note, only about 10% of patients had received prior adjuvant 5-FU treatment. Concerning the main endpoint of this study, the median TTP was statistically significantly longer with the combination than with 5-FU/FA alone (7.0 vs. 4.3 months; unstratified log-rank test, $p = 0.004$). This difference remained significant ($p = 0.002$) when a stratified log-rank test was applied. When adjusted for significant prognostic factors in a multivariate analysis, treatment with irinotecan/5-FU/FA remained a significant factor for TTP with a hazard ratio of 0.64 (95%, CI: 0.51–0.79). The median TTP with irinotecan alone was 4.2 months. The treatment with the irinotecan-containing combination was also associated with a statistically higher confirmed objective response rate (39 vs. 21%; $p = 0.0001$) compared with 5-FU/FA alone and with a statistically longer TTF . The objective response rate with irinotecan alone was 18%. Of note, also the median survival time with irinotecan/5-FU/FA was significantly longer than with 5-FU/FA alone (14.8 vs. 12.6 months; $p = 0.042$). When accounting for the impact of significant prognostic factors such as baseline LDH, performance status, white blood count, extent of organ involvement and total bilirubin in a multiple regression analysis, irinotecan/5-FU/FA treatment was again significantly correlated with improved survival with a p-value of 0.037. The median survival with irinotecan alone was 12.0 months. Summarizing the efficacy data, irinotecan/5-FU/FA was statistically significantly superior to 5-FU/FA with respect to TTP, TTF, response rate, and survival. Single-agent irinotecan and the conventional 5-FU/FA regimen were similar in terms of response rates, median TTP, median TTF, and median overall survival. Grade 3 and 4 diarrhea was seen in 23% of patients in the irinotecan/5-FU/FA arm and in 13% in the 5-FU/FA arm. The highest incidence of severe diarrhea (grade 3 and 4) was seen with irinotecan alone (31%). On the other hand, 5-FU/FA alone showed a significantly higher incidence of grade 4 neutropenia (42%) compared with either irinotecan/5-FU/FA (24%) or irinotecan alone (12%). Furthermore, neutropenic fever and mucositis were also seen more frequently in the 5-FU/FA arm. Quality of life was assessed during treatment with the EORTC QLQ C30. It could be demonstrated that treatment with the combination of irinotecan/5-FU/FA had no detrimental effect on overall quality of life and global health status compared with 5-FU/FA or irinotecan alone.

In the second multinational, multicentric randomized trial (study V 303) conducted in Europe and South Africa an infusional schedule of 5-FU was used [56]. This 5-FU/FA schedule was either the weekly 24-hour infusion of 5-FU in combination with high-dose FA (500 mg/m^2) (modified AIO regimen) or the biweekly De Gramont bolus and infusional regimen. Participating centers had to choose one of the two schedules. Depending on the 5-FU/FA schedule, irinotecan was given in the experimental treatment arm either in a dose of 80 mg/m^2 weekly ×6 in association with the AIO schedule (5-FU 2.3 g/m^2; FA 500 mg/m^2) or in a dose of 180 mg/m^2 every 2 weeks together with the De Gramont schedule. Except for the time since completion of adjuvant 5-FU treatment (> 6 months) and except for permitting prior pelvic irradiation, the study entry criteria were the same as in the Saltz trial. The main endpoint of study V 303 was response rate with the assumption that the combination of irinotecan/5-FU/FA would be associated with a 40% improvement in response rate and it was estimated that at least 169 patients per study arm were required to meet the study objectives. Secondary endpoints were TTP, TTF , overall survival, safety, and quality of life. Altogether 387 patients previously untreated with chemotherapy (other than adjuvant) for advanced CRC were accrued into this trial (5-FU/FA alone group: n = 188; irinotecan/5-FU/FA group: n = 199) from May 1997 to February 1998. Two patients (one in each arm) received no treatment because consent was withdrawn and were not included in the efficacy analysis. Approximately 25% of patients were randomized to the AIO regimens and approximately 75% to the De Gramont regimens. There was a good balance for known risk factors with the exception of a slight excess of rectal primaries in the combination arm. A higher proportion of patients than in the American trial had received prior adjuvant chemotherapy (25 vs. 10%, respectively). For the intention-to-treat population the confirmed response rates were 35% for the combination and 21% for the 5-FU/FA alone arm. This difference was statistically significant with a p-value of less than 0.005. In the response-evaluable population, the response rate was 49% for the combination and 31% for 5-FU/FA ($p < 0.001$) The time to tumor progression results also showed a statistically highly significant difference in favor of the combination treatment (6.7 vs. 4.4 months; $p < 0.001$). When TTP was compared with a stratified log-rank test including the four stratification factors, the results were also statistically significant ($p = 0.002$). This was still true when adjusted by the Cox regression process for prognostic factors such as involved organ sites and baseline serum LDH. The hazard ratio indicates a 41% reduction in the risk of progression. A survival advantage for early combination therapy with irinotecan/5-FU/FA was confirmed in study V 303. The median survival time with combination treatment was 17.4 months versus 14.1 months among those patients randomized to 5-FU/FA only. When comparing this difference using the unstratified log-rank test, the result was statistically significant with a p-value of 0.032. Again, when considering prognostic factors, irinotecan/5-FU/FA treatment was significantly correlated to improved survival ($p = 0.045$). The response analysis by regimen showed overall responses of 51 and 38% for the weekly-times-six and for the biweekly regimen, respectively, using the combination of irinotecan and 5-FU/FA. The weekly and biweekly 5-FU/FA regimens alone produced 29 and 21% overall responses, respectively. Concerning toxicities, a higher incidence of neutropenia grade 3 and 4 occurred with the combination (42 vs. 11%, $p < 0.01$), however, this did not result in a significantly higher rate of neutropenic fever or infection. Severe diarrhea (grade 3 and 4) was less frequent with 5-FU/FA alone (10%) compared with the combination treatment (22%). As in the US study, the addition of irinotecan to 5-FU/FA had no negative impact on the overall health status and quality of life.

Based on the results of these two studies it can be concluded that the addition of irinotecan to 5-FU/FA resulted in a significantly longer TTP, progression-free survival and, especially noteworthy, also in a significantly longer survival time as well as in a significantly higher objective response rate without impairing quality of life. Therefore, the combination of irinotecan with 5-FU/FA has to be considered as a new standard first-line treatment for patients with metastatic CRC.

Summary

The recent developments that have been made in the past years clearly show that chemotherapy of advanced, metastatic CRC is a clinically meaningful approach as first-line therapy as well as salvage therapy. In that context, irinotecan in combination chemotherapy is an important step forward in the management of CRC and contributes to an improved prognosis of this disease.

References

1 The Advanced Colorectal Cancer Meta-Analysis Project: Modulation of fluorouracil by leucovorin in patients with advanced colorectal cancer: Evidence in terms of response. J Clin Oncol 1992;10: 896–903.

2 Köhne CH, Schöffski P, Wilke H, et al: Effective biomodulation by leucovorin of high-dose infusion fluorouracil given as a weekly 24-hour infusion: Results of a randomized trial in patients with advanced colorectal cancer. J Clin Oncol 1998;16: 418–426.

3 De Gramont A, Bosset JF, Milan C, Rougier P, Bouche O, Etienne PL, Morvan F, Louvet C, Guillot T, Francois E, Bedenne L: Randomized trial comparing monthly low-dose leucovorin and fluorouracil bolus with bimonthly high-dose leucovorin and fluorouracil bolus plus continuous infusion for advanced colorectal cancer. J Clin Oncol 1997;15: 808–815.

4 Chen AY, Liu LF: DNA topoisomerases: Essential enzymes and lethal targets. Annu Rev Pharmacol Toxicol 1994;34:191–218.

5 Lavelle F, Bissery MC, André S, et al: Preclinical evaluation of CPT-11 and its active metabolite SN-38. Semin Oncol 1996;23(suppl 3):11–20.

6 Pommier Y: Eukaryotic DNA topoisomerase I: Genome gatekeeper and its intruders, camptothecins. Semin Oncol 1996;23(suppl 3):3–10.

7 Wisemann LR, Markham A: Irinotecan: A review of its pharmacological properties and clinical efficacy in the management of advanced colorectal cancer. Drugs 1996;52:606–623.

8 Conti JA, Kemeny NE, Saltz LB, et al: Irinotecan is an active agent in untreated patients with metastatic colorectal cancer. J Clin Oncol 1996;14:709–715.

9 Pitot HC, Wender DB, O'Connell MJ, et al: Phase II trial of irinotecan in patients with metastatic colorectal carcinoma. J Clin Oncol 1997;8:2910–2919.

10 Rougier P, Bugat R, Douillard JY, et al: Phase II study of irinotecan in the treatment of advanced colorectal cancer in chemotherapy-naïve patients and patients pretreated with fluorouracil-based chemotherapy. J Clin Oncol 1997;15:251–260.

11 Irigoyen AL, Firvida JL, Vazquez S, et al: Phase II trial of irinotecan (CPT-11) in patients with not pretreated advanced colorectal cancer. Proc Am Soc Clin Oncol 1998;17:279a(abstr).

12 Pozzo C, Pyrhönen S, Bodrogi I, et al: A randomized phase II trial assessing irinotecan (IRI) and 5FU/folinic acid (LV), 'Mayo regimen', in first line palliative chemotherapy patients with metastatic colorectal cancer. Eur J Cancer 1999;35(suppl 4): S70(abstr).

13 Saltz LB, Locker PK, Pirotta N, et al: Weekly irinotecan (CPT-11), leucovorin (LV), and fluorouracil (FU) is superior to daily x5 LV/FU in patients with previously untreated metastatic colorectal cancer. Proc Am Soc Clin Oncol 1999;18: 233a(abstr).

14 Van Cutsem E, Rougier P, Droz JP, et al: Clinical benefit of irinotecan (CPT-11) in metastatic colorectal cancer resistant to 5-FU. Proc Am Soc Clin Oncol 1997;16:268a(abstr).

15 Rothenberg ML, Hainsworth JD, Rosen L, et al: Phase II study of irinotecan (CPT-11) 250 mg/m^2 given every-other-week in previously treated colorectal cancer patients. Proc Am Soc Clin Oncol 1998;17:284a(abstr).

16 Van Cutsem E, Cunningham D, Ten Bokkel Huinink WW, et al: Clinical activity and benefit of irinotecan (CPT-11) in patients with colorectal cancer truly resistant to 5-fluorouracil (5-FU). Eur J Cancer 1999;35:54–59.

17 Tsavaris N, Polyzos A, Georgoulias V, et al: Irinotecan (CPT-11) in patients with advanced colon carcinoma (ACC) relapsing after 5-fluorouracil (5-FU)-leucovorin (LV) combination. Proc Am Soc Clin Oncol 1998;17:304a(abstr).

18 Anton A, Aranda E, Carrato A, et al: Phase II study of irinotecan (CPT-11) in the treatment of patients with advanced colorectal cancer resistant to 5-fluorouracil (5-FU) based chemotherapy. The experience of TTD Spanish Cooperative Group. Proc Am Soc Clin Oncol 1998;17:278a(abstr).

19 Frontini L, Labianca R, Sobrero A, et al: Irinotecan (CPT-11) is effective as second-line chemotherapy in advanced colorectal cancer: A phase II trial of GISCAD (Italian Group for the Study of Gastrointestinal Cancer). Proc Am Soc Clin Oncol 1999;18: 260a(abstr).

20 Hoeffken K, Ridwelsky C, Wein A, et al: Phase II study of irinotecan as second line chemotherapy in metastatic colorectal cancer. Proc Am Soc Clin Oncol 1999;18:244a(abstr).

21 Santoro A, Santoro M, Maiorino L, et al: Irinotecan (CPT-11) in patients with 5-FU refractory metastatic colorectal carcinoma. Proc Am Soc Clin Oncol 1999;18:251a(abstr).

22 Vicent JM, Aparicio J, Lizon J, et al: 5-FU-highly resistant advanced colorectal cancer patients treated with CPT-11. A phase II trial. Proc Am Soc Clin Oncol 1999;18:303a(abstr).

23 Rothenberg ML, Eckardt JR, Kuhn JG, et al: Phase II trial of irinotecan in patients with progressive or rapidly recurrent colorectal cancer. J Clin Oncol 1996;14:1128–1135.

24 Rothenberg ML, Cox JV, Russell F, et al: A multicenter, phase II trial of weekly irinotecan (CPT-11) in patients with previously treated colorectal carcinoma. Cancer 1999;85:786–795.

25 Michael M, Moore MJ, Hedley D, et al: A phase II study of irinotecan (CPT-11) as palliative therapy in refractory advanced colorectal cancer. Proc Am Soc Clin Oncol 1999;18:243a(abstr).

26 Cunningham D, Pyrhönen S, James RD, et al: Randomised trial of irinotecan plus supportive care versus supportive care alone after fluorouracil failure for patients with metastatic colorectal cancer. Lancet 1998;352:1413–1418.

27 Rougier P, Van Cutsem E, Bajetta E, et al: Randomised trial of irinotecan versus fluorouracil by continuous infusion after fluorouracil failure in patients with metastatic colorectal cancer. Lancet 1998;352:1407–1412.

28 Aranda E, Carrato A, Cervantes A, et al: Phase I/II study of escalating doses of weekly irinotecan (CPT-11) in combination with 5-fluorouracil (5-FU) (48 h continuous i.v. infusion) in patients with advanced solid tumors. Proc Am Soc Clin Oncol 1999;18:277a(abstr).

29 Benhammouda A, Bastian G, Rixe O, et al: A phase I and pharmacokinetic study of CPT-11 and 5-FU in combination. Proc Am Soc Clin Oncol 1997;16:202a(abstr).

30 Comella P, Casaretti R, De Vita F, et al: Concurrent irinotecan and 5-fluorouracil plus levo-folinic acid given every other week in the first-line management of advanced colorectal carcinoma: A phase I study of the Southern Italy Cooperative Oncology Group. Ann Oncol 1999;10:915–921.

31 Ducreux M, Ychou M, Seitz JF, et al: Irinotecan combined with bolus fluorouracil, continuous infusion fluorouracil, and high-dose leucovorin every two weeks (LV5FU2 regimen): A clinical dose-finding and pharmacokinetic study in patients with pretreated metastatic colorectal cancer. J Clin Oncol 1999;17:2901–2908.

32 Falcone A, Danesi R, Allegrini G, et al: Escalating dose irinotecan (CPT-11) immediately prior or after 5-fluorouracil (5-FU) 48 hours infusion + leucovorin (LV): Pharmacokinetic and pharmacodynamic interactions in chemotherapy-naïve metastatic colorectal cancer patients. Proc Am Soc Clin Oncol 1999;18:241a(abstr).

33 Fonseca R, Goldberg RM, Erlichman C, et al: Phase I study of the combination of CPT-11/5-FU and leucovorin (LV). Proc Am Soc Clin Oncol 1998;17:203a(abstr).

34 Garufi C, Tampellini M, D'Attino RM, et al: A phase I study of CPT-11 plus chrono-modulated (chrono) 5-fluorouracil (5-FU) and l-folinic acid (FA) in advanced colorectal cancer patients. Third International Conference on Biology, Prevention and Treatment of Gastrointestinal Malignancies, 1998, Cologne, Germany.
35 Kakolyris S, Androulakis N, Souglakos J, et al: Phase I study with irinotecan (CPT-11) plus 5-fluorouracil (5-FU; 4-DY C.I.) combination in advanced colon cancer. Proc Am Soc Clin Oncol 1998;17:278a(abstr).
36 Saltz LB, Kanowitz J, Kemeny NE, et al: Phase I clinical and pharmacokinetic study of irinotecan, fluorouracil, and leucovorin in patients with advanced solid tumors. J Clin Oncol 1996;14:2959–2967.
37 Sastre H, Paz-Ares L, Diaz-Rubio E, et al: Phase I dose finding study of irinotecan (CPT-11) over a short IV infusion combined with a fixed dose of 5-fluorouracil (5-FU) over a protracted IV infusion in patients with advanced solid tumors. Proc Am Soc Clin Oncol 1998;17:201a(abstr).
38 Vanhoefer U, Harstrick A, Köhne CH, et al: Phase I study of a weekly schedule of irinotecan, high-dose leucovorin, and infusional fluorouracil as first-line chemotherapy in patients with advanced colorectal cancer. J Clin Oncol 1999;17:907–913.
39 Vanhoefer U, Harstrick A, Achterrath W, et al: Extended phase I study of a weekly schedule of irinotecan (CPT-11), leucovorin and infusional 5-FU as first-line chemotherapy in metastatic colorectal cancer. Clin Cancer Res 1999;5(suppl): 3799s(abstr).
40 Falcone A, Allegrini G, Masi G, et al: Irinotecan in combination with leucovorin and 5-fluorouracil 48 hours continuous infusion: A phase I study with pharmacokinetic, DNA damage and topoisomerase I/DNA complexes evaluation in chemotherapy naïve metastatic colorectal cancer patients. Proc Am Soc Clin Oncol 1998;17:290a(abstr).
41 Ford HER, Cunningham D, Ross PJ, et al: Open label dose finding phase I study of irinotecan hydrochloride and raltitrexed in patients with advanced gastrointestinal tract adenocarcinoma. Proc Am Soc Clin Oncol 1999;18:176a(abstr).
42 Sun W, Stevenson JP, Gallagher M, et al: Phase I and pharmacokinetic trial of irinotecan (CPT-11) and tomudex administered as sequential IV infusions, D1 and D2, repeated every 21 days. Clin Cancer Res 1999;5(suppl):3799s(abstr).
43 Goldwasser F, Gross M, Tigaud JM, et al: CPT-11/oxaliplatin (L-OHP) combination every two weeks: Final results of a phase I study in advanced digestive malignancies. Proc Am Soc Clin Oncol 1999;18:176a(abstr).
44 Rothenberg ML, McKinney J, Hande KR, et al: A phase I clinical and pharmacokinetic trial of oxaliplatin and irinotecan (CPT-11) given every two weeks to patients with refractory solid tumors. Clin Cancer Res 1999;5(suppl):3853s(abstr).
45 Wasserman E, Cuvier E, Lokiec F, et al: Combination of oxaliplatin plus irinotecan in patients with gastrointestinal tumors: Results of two independent phase I studies with pharmacokinetics. J Clin Oncol 1999;17:1751–1759.
46 Rothenberg ML, Pazdur R, Rowinsky EK, et al: A phase II multicenter trial of alternating cycles of irinotecan (CPT-11) and 5-FU/LV in patients with previously untreated metastatic colorectal cancer. Proc Am Soc Clin Oncol 1997;18:266a(abstr).
47 Van Cutsem E, Pozzo C, Starkhammar H, et al: A phase II study of irinotecan alternated with five days bolus of 5-fluorouracil and leucovorin in first-line chemotherapy of metastatic colorectal cancer. Ann Oncol 1998;9:1199–1204.
48 Kalbakis K, Kandylis N, Stavrakakis J, et al: First line chemotherapy with 5-fluorouracil (5-FU), leucovorin (LV) and irinotecan (CPT-11) in advanced colorectal cancer: A multicenter phase II study. Proc Am Soc Clin Oncol 1999;18:257a(abstr).
49 Lipp R, Hegewichs-Becker S, Göthert J, et al: Decrease of severe toxicities by reducing the 5-FU-dosage in the combination therapy with CPT-11/5-FU/FA weekly in patients with advanced colorectal cancer. Onkologie 1999;22(suppl 1):84(abstr).
50 Graeven U, Ridwelski K, Manns M, et al: Irinotecan (CPT-11) with bolus 5-fluorouracil (5-FU) and folinic acid (FA) in patients with previously untreated metastatic colorectal cancer: An active and safe regimen. Proc Am Soc Clin Oncol 2000;19: (submitted for publication).
51 Maiello E, Giuliani F, Gebbia V, et al: Folinic acid (FA) and 5-fluorouracil /FU) alone or with irinotecan (CPT-11) for advanced colorectal cancer: Preliminary results of a randomized phase II trial. Eur J Cancer 1999;35(suppl 4):220(abstr).
52 Andre T, Léuvet C, Maindrault-Goebel F, et al: CPT-11 (irinotecan) addition to bimonthly, high-dose leucovorin and bolus and continuous-infusion 5-fluorouracil (FOLFIRI) for pretreated metastatic colorectal cancer. Eur J Cancer 1999;35:1343–1347.
53 Duranni ASK, Benhammouda A, Gil-Delgado MA, et al: Combination of irinotecan with leucovorin and 5-FU in advanced colorectal carcinoma – a phase II study. Proc Am Soc Clin Oncol 1999;18: 282a(abstr).
54 Scheithauer W, Kornek GV, Raderer M, et al: Combined irinotecan and oxaliplatin plus granulocyte colony-stimulating factor in patients with advanced fluoropyrimidine/leucovorin-pretreated colorectal cancer. J Clin Oncol 1999;17:902–906.
55 Scheithauer W, Kornek GV, Brugger S, et al: Randomized phase II study of irinotecan plus mitomycin (MMC) versus oxaliplatin plus MMC in patients with advanced fluoropyrimidine/leucovorin-pretreated colorectal cancer (ACC). Onkologie 1999;22(suppl 1):78(abstr).
56 Douillard JY, Cunningham D, Roth AD, et al: Irinotecan combined with fluorouracil compared with fluorouracil alone as first-line treatment for metastatic colorectal cancer: A multicentre randomised trial. Lancet 2000;355:1041–1047.

ONKOLOGIE

Onkologie 2000;23(suppl 4):15–17

Irinotecan in Second-Line Therapy of Metastatic Colorectal Cancer

E. Jäger D. Jäger J. Orth A. Knuth

Medizinische Klinik II, Krankenhaus Nordwest, Frankfurt/Main

Modern cytostatic chemotherapy makes use of a wide range of drugs with variable antineoplastic effects. Alkylating agents, antimetabolites, mitosis inhibitors, antibiotics, and enzyme inhibitors are most commonly used. The cytostatic effect of these drugs is attributable to the inhibition of cell division and metabolism at different levels. The clinical treatment results could, theoretically, be improved by combining cytostatic drugs that have different effects. The antineoplastic efficacy of a given drug therapy in relation to its toxicity is especially good when a tumor-associated molecular structure or metabolic function can be defined as the target. The enzyme topoisomerase I was defined as a potential target structure in the 1970s. This enzyme is responsible for opening and closing the DNA double helix during physiological transcriptional and regulatory processes. Inhibition of topoisomerase I results in an interruption of DNA synthesis, thereby inhibiting cell division.

Irinotecan, a semisynthetic topoisomerase I inhibitor, is a so-called 'prodrug' derived from an alkaloid of the Asian *Camptotheca acuminata* plant. After being metabolized with hepatic carboxylesterases, the substance is transformed to 7-ethyl-10-hydroxycamptothecin, which is 100 times more potent than the prodrug. The metabolized product binds to the topoisomerase-enzyme complex. This inhibits the closure of the opened DNA double helix, resulting in irreversible DNA strand breakage and cell death. Since a selective increase in topoisomerase I expression occurs in tumor tissues, especially in colon cancer, the selective activity of the topoisomerase I inhibitors unfolds primarily within the tumor tissue.

A number of clinical studies in a cumulative total of more than 1500 patients with colon cancer have convincingly demonstrated the efficacy of irinotecan in primary antineoplastic therapy; the drug also proved effective in second-line therapy after failure of the standard 5-fluorouracil regimen. Irinotecan has achieved remission rates of 18–20% for a mean duration of 9 months when used as the primary drug in phase II studies [1].

Based on these promising phase II studies two randomized trials in second-line therapy were conducted: One compared best supportive care (BSC) with a treatment arm adding irinotecan (350 mg/m^2 every 3 weeks) to BSC [2]. 279 patients with failure of a 5-FU-based therapy regimen were randomized (2:1) for irinotecan or BSC. Aim of this study was to answer the question whether patients will profit from a second-line treatment. After one year 36.2% of the patients in the irinotecan group were alive but only 13.8% in the BSC group ($p = 0.00001$). The median survival was 2.7 months longer in the irinotecan arm. The clinical benefit was also significant. In terms of survival without weight loss, survival without performance deterioration, pain-free survival and quality of life, there was a clear advantage for the irinotecan treatment arm. Drug-related toxicity was manageable, with 21% diarrhea (grade 3, 4), 22% neutropenia, 14% nausea and vomiting. Interestingly, the asthenia rate in the BSC arm was higher than in the treatment arm (15 vs. 19%). The authors concluded from these results that there is a clear advantage in terms of survival, quality of life and other clinical parameters for a second-line treatment with irinotecan (fig. 1).

The second study compared ironotecan (350 mg/m^2 every 3 weeks) with the 'best estimated 5-FU/FA infusional regimen' [3]. From a total of 267 patients, 133 were randomized for irinotecan and 134 for 5-FU. About 20–30% of the patients had already a 5-FU infusional regimen as prior therapy. One out of three different 5-FU-schedules could be chosen by the study center: De Gramont, Lokich or AIO (ratio: 35:39:55). The primary objective in this study was survival. As in the above-mentioned study there was a survival advantage for patients treated with irinotecan. The survival probability after 6, 9 and 12 months with irinotecan was 78, 63 and 45%, and that in the 5-FU arm was 65, 47 and 45%, respectively. The median survival time was 10.8 with irintocan and 8.5 months with 5-FU. The median progression-free survival was also prolonged in the irinotecan group with 4.2 vs. 2.9 months. The difference in side-effect profile did not result in a difference in quality of

KARGER

Fax +49 761 4 52 07 14
E-mail Information@Karger.de
www.karger.com

Accessible online at:
www.karger.com/journals/onk

Prof. Dr. A. Knuth
II. Medizinische Klinik
Krankenhaus Nordwest
Steinbacher Hohl 2–26
D-60488 Frankfurt/Main (Germany)

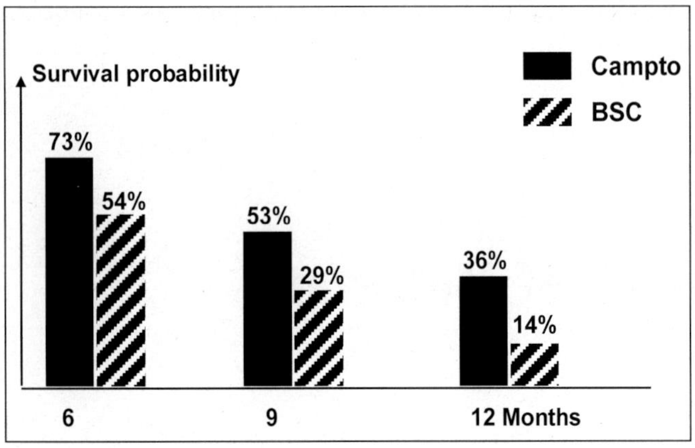

Fig. 1. Probability of survival after treatment with ironotecan and best supportive care (BSC).

life; this was comparable in both treatment arms. The incidence of severe diarrhea was with 22% also lower than in former studies.

These results showed that a second-line therapy with irinotecan influences survival and quality of life in patients with colorectal cancer.

In light of these encouraging data, irinotecan has first been approved and recommended for second-line treatment of metastatic colorectal cancer. Since irinotecan has been found to have a higher rate of toxicity than the standard treatment with 5-fluorouracil [5], especially with regards to hematotoxicity and gastrointestinal side effects, a modified treatment scheme has now been clinically tested. For example, 100–125 mg/m^2 of irinotecan is administered once weekly as compared to the higher doses of the monthly administration scheme (350–400 mg/m^2 once every 3 weeks).

The efficacy of irinotecan combined with 5-fluorouracil at various dose levels is also being investigated. Results from randomized studies of irinotecan/5-fluorouracil/folinic acid versus 5-fluorouracil/folinic acid (versus irinotecan alone) have shown that the results with the irinotecan/5-fluorouracil/folinic combination were clearly superior to those of 5-fluorouracil/folinic acid and irinotecan alone with respect to the remission rate, progression-free intervals, and overall survival [4, 6]. Ongoing studies are now investigating the question of whether modification of the dose and/or time of irinotecan administration (every 3 weeks versus weekly therapy) in conjunction with 5-fluorouracil/folinic acid administration (24-hour infusion versus 5-day rhythm) can affect the clinical efficacy of treatment with respect to the rate of remission, progression-free interval, and toxicity.

The primary goals of palliative treatment regimens, especially for colorectal cancer, have been redefined and often debated over the past 10 years. The remission rate was considered to be the primary criterion in the 1980s. Some very toxic combination chemotherapy regimens were used to achieve as high a remission rate as possible. However, this did not help to extend the overall survival time, and the treatment significantly detracted from the patients' quality of life. As a result, the variables 'quality of life' and 'progression-free interval' are now being more heavily weighted, even in patients in whom treatment cannot be expected to achieve any objectively discernible tumor reduction. Investigators have shown that the tumor-related complaints associated with palliative treatment measures can be improved, even in cases where no measurable reduction in tumor mass occurs. In addition, randomized studies have shown that, compared to purely supportive measures, palliative chemotherapy significantly extends the overall survival time and improves the quality of life, provided the level of treatment-related toxicity is low [7]. Considering the findings with irinotecan and the value of palliative treatment of colorectal cancer, the ongoing studies will address the following questions.

1. Can second-line therapy with irinotecan alone or in combination with 5-fluorouracil/folinic acid significantly extend the progression-free intervals and overall survival time at a tolerable level of toxicity?
2. Can first-line therapy with irinotecan alone or in combination with 5-fluorouracil/folinic acid significantly improve the treatment results and extend the overall survival time, thus providing a regimen that can be recommended for primary treatment of metastatic colorectal cancer?

Extending the survival time while maintaining a high quality of life is the primary goal of treatment strategies to improve the overall prognosis of patients with metastatic colorectal carcinoma. It may be possible to extend the overall survival time by performing sequential palliative measures. One study showed that, after failure of weekly 5-fluorouracil/folinic acid therapy, a renewed response could be achieved by raising the 5-fluorouracil dose, and that second-line therapy achieved a 24% remission rate at a low level of toxicity [8]. Future studies should be designed to investigate the therapeutic efficacy of treatment protocols using irinotecan in a larger context of different but coordinated steps of therapy. Considering the current status of information on the efficacy of first- and second-line therapy with irinotecan, it would appear prudent to perform different studies, such as a randomized study of irinotecan alone versus the drug combination, while using a protocol in which the 5-fluorouracil dose is modified at various increments. Such protocols are already available, and the corresponding studies have been initiated.

Experimental clinical treatment concepts hold further perspectives for the use of irinotecan. Other 'new' drugs for treatment of colorectal cancer, such as oxaliplatin, capecitabine, and raltitrexed, have achieved encouraging results in phase II studies. It may be possible to improve upon the previous results by combining these drugs with irinotecan, provided the treatment-related toxicity remains at an acceptable level for palliative treatment.

The experimental concept of whole-body hyperthermia concomitant with cytostatic chemotherapy is also gaining more and more recognition. A phase I study combining irinotecan with whole-body hyperthermia has been planned for patients with progression of colorectal cancer after primary therapy with 5-fluorouracil. However, it is not yet possible to assess the value of whole-body hyperthermia in this indication.

Strategies for passive immunotherapy with monoclonal antibodies (A33, 17–1A, F-19) are currently being evaluated in patients with metastatic colorectal cancer [9]. Although phase I/II studies using passive immunotherapeutic strategies have not achieved higher remission rates than those using palliative chemotherapy, very long progression-free intervals have been achieved in some cases. This is an important indication of the clinical efficacy of antibody therapy. It may be possible to effectively enhance the action of monoclonal antibodies via complementary cytostatic chemotherapy. Hence, the inclusion of irinotecan in the framework of phase I studies is a fundamental perspective for treatment concepts based on monoclonal antibodies.

References

1 Rougier P, Bugat R, Douillard JY, Culine S, Suc E, Brunet P, Becouarn Y, Ychou M, Marty M, Extra JM, Bonneterre J, Adenis A, Seitz JF, Ganem G, Namer M, Conroy T, Negrier S, Merrouche Y, Burki F, Mousseau M, Herait P, Mahjoubi M: Phase II study of irinotecan in the treatment of advanced colorectal cancer in chemotherapy-naive patients and patients pretreated with fluorouracil-based chemotherapy. J Clin Oncol 1997;15:251–260.

2 Cunningham D, Pyrhönen S, James R D, Punt CJA, Hickish T F, Heikkila R, Johannesen T B, Starkammar H, Topham C A, Awad L, Jacques C, Herait P: Randomised trial of irinotecan plus supportive care versus supportive care alone after fluorouracil failure for patients with metastatic colorectal cancer. Lancet 1998;352:1413–1418.

3 Rougier P, Van Cutsem E, Bajetta E, Niederle N, Possinger K, Labianca R, Navarro M, Morant R, Bleiberg H, Wils J, Awad L, Herait P, Jacques C: Randomised trial of irinotecan versus fluorouracil by continuous infusion after fluorouracil failure in patients with metastatic colorectal cancer. Lancet 1998;352:1407–1412.

4 Douillard JY, Cunningham D, Roth AD, Navarro M, James RD, Karasek P, Jandik P, Jueson T, Carmichael J, Alaki M, Gruia G, Awad L, Rangier P: Ironotecan combined with fluorouracil compared with fluorouracil alone as first-line treatment for metastatic colorectal cancer: A multicentre randomised trial. Lancet 2000;355:1041–1043.

5 Saliba F, Hagipantelli R, Misset JL, Bastian G, Vassal G, Bonnay M, Herait P, Cote C, Mahjoubi M, Mignard D, Cvitkovic E: Pathophysiology and therapy of irinotecan-induced delayed-onset diarrhea in patients with advanced colorectal cancer: a prospective assessment. J Clin Oncol 1998;16: 2745–2751.

6 Salz LB, Locker PK, Pirotta N, Elfring GL, Miller LL: Weekly irinotecan (CPT-11), leucovorin (LV), and fluorouracil (FU) is superior to daily x5 LV/FU in patients (pts) with previously untreated metastatic colorectal cancer (CRC). Proc Am Soc Clin Oncol 1999;18.

7 Scheithauer W, Rosen H, Kornek GV, Sebesta C, Depisch D: Randomised comparison of combination chemotherapy plus supportive care with supportive care alone in patients with metastatic colorectal cancer. Br Med J 1993;306:752–755.

8 Jager E, Klein O, Wächter B, Muller B, Braun U, Knuth A: High dose 5-fluorouracil (5-FU) and folinic acid in advanced colorectal cancer resistant to standard dose 5-FU treatment: results of a phase II study. Eur J Cancer 1995;31A:1717.

9 Welt S, Scott AM, Divgi CR, Kemeny NE, Finn RD, Daghighian F, Germain JS, Richards EC, Larson SM, Old LJ: Phase I/II study of iodine 125-labeled monoclonal antibody A33 in patients with advanced colon cancer. J Clin Oncol 1996;14: 1787–1797.

ONKOLOGIE

Onkologie 2000;23(suppl 4):18–22

Campto® – Strategies for Adjuvant and Neoadjuvant Chemotherapy of Colorectal Cancer

R. Lipp

Abteilung Onkologie und Hämatologie, Medizinische Klinik, Universitätskrankenhaus Eppendorf, Hamburg

Introduction

Clinical studies performed in the USA and Europe within the past 3 years have shown that the combination chemotherapy regimen of CPT-11 (Campto®, irinotecan) plus 5-fluorouracil (5-FU) and folinic acid (FA) achieves a significantly better response and survival than 5-FU/FA alone in patients with metastatic or progressive colorectal cancer [5, 20]. In light of these findings, other interesting indications for CPT-11 + 5-FU/FA in colorectal cancer are now being researched. Because of its proven high antitumor activity, as reflected by response rates of 49–75% [5, 11, 20, 21], this combination chemotherapy regimen holds promise for other indications, especially adjuvant and neoadjuvant chemotherapy.

Previous Standard Treatment Regimens

Combination chemotherapy regimens using 5-FU and FA are still considered to be the standard regimens for *adjuvant therapy* of patients with Dukes C (UICC stage III) colorectal cancer. The so-called 'Mayo Clinic scheme' (5-FU: 425 mg/m^2 i.v. on days 1–5, FA: 20 mg/m^2 i.v. on days 1–5, repeated every 28 days for 6 months) is the regimen most commonly used in Germany. When administered for adjuvant chemotherapy after complete tumor resection, this regimen has achieved significant increases in the 5-year survival and significant decreases in the risk of tumor recurrence compared to tumor resection alone [7–9, 14–16, 18, 22]. The Mayo Clinic scheme is now being compared with a weekly continuous infusion regimen (PETACC2 study) in a larger scale clinical study of adjuvant chemotherapy regimens. The final results of this study are not in yet.
None of the leading medical societies have yet recommended a standard adjuvant chemotherapy regimen for Dukes B (UICC stage II) colorectal carcinoma. A large-scale American retrospective meta-analysis found that adjuvant chemotherapy has a beneficial effect on patient survival [13], but a European analysis did not find any such benefits [7]. Hence, further investigations are currently being performed to clear up these controversies.
After *resection of hepatic metastases* from colorectal tumors, 35% of the patients survive another 5 years without further treatment, but 60% develop tumor recurrences within 2 years [3]. Various systemic and regional polychemotherapy regimens have been tested to determine the efficacy of 5-FU and its derivatives for adjuvant treatment after the resection of hepatic metastases [1, 4, 6, 9, 10, 12, 19]. However, only a few isolated studies have revealed a positive effect on patient survival [9, 10]. As a result, none of the respective societies have yet recommended a standard adjuvant chemotherapy regimen for use after the resection of metastases.
Regarding *neoadjuvant chemotherapy*, Bismuth et al. [2] showed that chronomodulated oxaliplatin + 5-FU/FA significantly increases patient survival if chemotherapy achieved complete resectability of hepatic metastases from colorectal carcinomas.
In the following sections, we will attempt to provide an overview of the ongoing clinical studies and of newly proposed strategies for the use of CPT-11 plus 5-FU/FA in chemotherapy. Special attention will be devoted to adjuvant chemotherapy of patients with Dukes B and C colorectal carcinomas, postoperative chemotherapy regimens after complete resection of liver metastases from colorectal carcinomas, and neoadjuvant chemotherapy of initially inoperable colorectal tumors.

Ongoing Clinical Studies of Campto plus 5-FU/FA in Adjuvant Chemotherapy

In Stage II and III (Dukes B and C) Colorectal Carcinomas
A number of studies have shown that the use of 5-FU/FA alone (bolus administration or short infusion) significantly in-

KARGER
Fax +49 761 4 52 07 14
E-mail Information@Karger.de
www.karger.com

Accessible online at:
www.karger.com/journals/onk

Dr. med. Rainer Lipp
Martinistraße 52
20246 Hamburg (Germany)

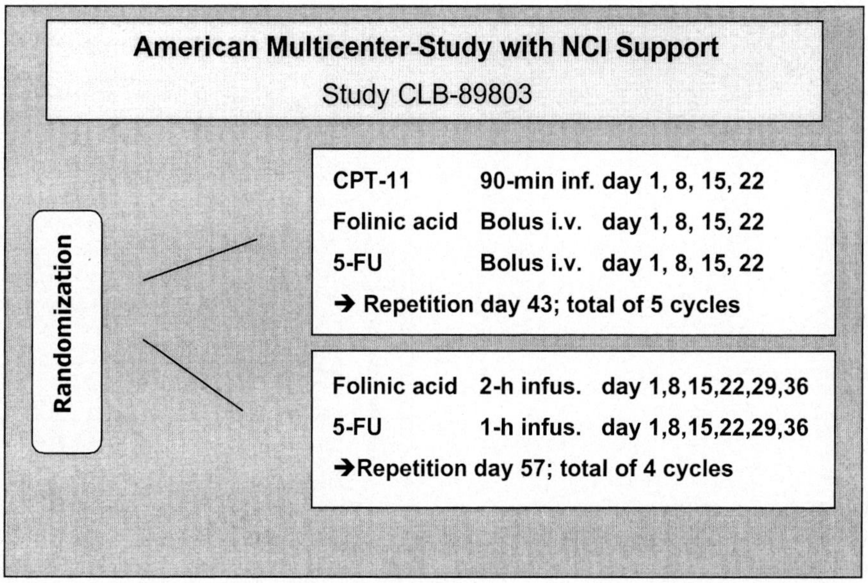

Fig. 1. Design of a North American study comparing CPT-11 + 5-FU/FA to 5-FU/FA alone in patients with Dukes C colorectal cancer.

creases long-term survival rates. However, combination chemotherapy with CPT-11 + 5-FU/FA was shown to have significantly better antitumor activity with increased survival than the aforementioned regimen in patients with advanced colorectal cancer [5, 11, 20, 22]. Several studies demonstrated that the regimen has very high antitumor activity, with response rates of 50–75% (partial and complete response). Therefore, the combination of CPT-11 plus 5-FU/FA can also be expected to achieve better results than 5-FU/FA alone in adjuvant chemotherapy. Large-scale multicenter studies will be performed to investigate these questions in patients with stage III (Dukes B) and, in some cases stage II (Dukes B) colorectal carcinomas.

In North America, a multicenter study of Cancer and Leukemia Group B (CLB) is being performed with the support of the NCI to compare the effects of combination chemotherapy with CPT-11 plus bolus i.v. doses of 5-FU and FA to chemotherapy with 5-FU and FA alone (fig. 1). The investigators plan to recruit 1260 patients with stage III (T_x, N_{1-2}, M_0) colorectal carcinomas in the next 3 years.

A similar large-scale multicenter study (RP 64174-V-307) was started in Europe in late 1999. The goal of the study is to compare the efficacy of combination chemotherapy with CPT-11 plus high-dose continuous infusions of 5-FU/FA with chemotherapy with high-dose 5-FU/FA alone in patients with stage III (Dukes C) colorectal carcinomas (see fig. 2 for study design). A total of 1800 patients are to be recruited for the study from more than 120 centers in over 25 European countries in the next few years. The combination of CPT-11 + 5-FU/FA is expected to improve the 3-year tumor-free survival by at least 7% as compared to 5-FU/FA alone. Considering the 2-year recruitment period, the first survival data can be expected around the year 2004. Parallel to the group of stage III patients, the investigators will also recruit an additional group of patients with stage II colorectal carcinomas (T_{3-4}, N_0, M_0) to determine if high-dose adjuvant chemotherapy is beneficial in this tumor stage (regional tumor spread without lymph node metastasis).

Comparable to the multicenter study of metastatic colorectal cancer, the participating study centers can also decide whether to administer the chemotherapy in biweekly cycles (De Gramont regimen) or weekly cycles (AIO and Ardalan regimens). The proposed duration of treatment is 6 months for both groups.

After Complete Resection of Liver Metastases from Colorectal Carcinomas

A number of investigators have already attempted to improve the rates of recurrence-free and long-term survival of patients with colorectal carcinomas by administering adjuvant chemotherapy after resection of hepatic metastases. These investigators mainly used systemic chemotherapy regimens with 5-FU and FA, but also used regional chemotherapy with 5-FU with or without FA administered by hepatic artery infusion, or they used combined regional and systemic chemotherapy. Some of the investigators found that adjuvant chemotherapy has a beneficial effect on recurrence-free or long-term survival [9, 10], whereas others found the effects of adjuvant regional chemotherapy to be worse than surgery alone [12]. Therefore, none of the surgical or oncological societies have yet issued any standard recommendations regarding adjuvant chemotherapy after the resection of colonic carcinoma metastases to the liver.

Combination chemotherapy with CPT-11 and 5-FU/FA has not yet been assessed in this indication. A German multicenter study (Study UKE 001) was therefore been initiated under

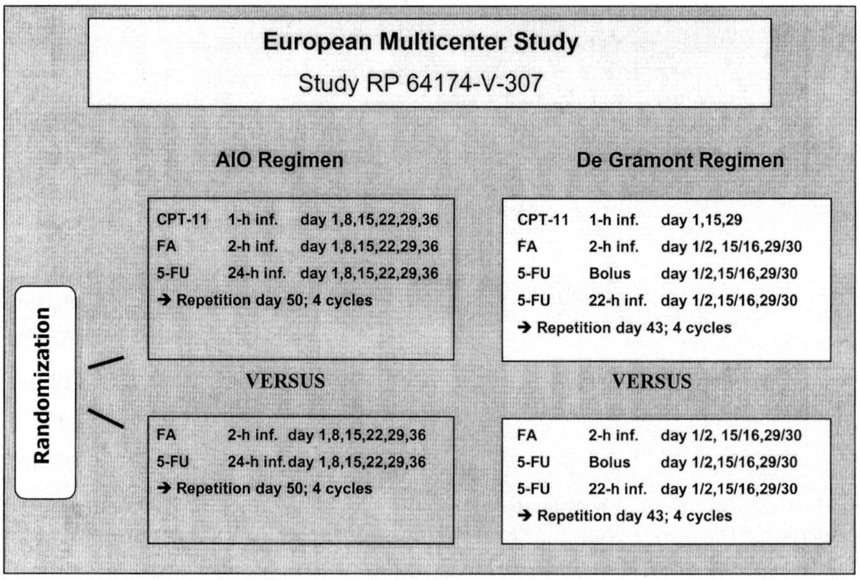

Fig. 2. Design of a European multicenter study on adjuvant chemotherapy of stage II/III (Dukes B and C) colorectal cancer.

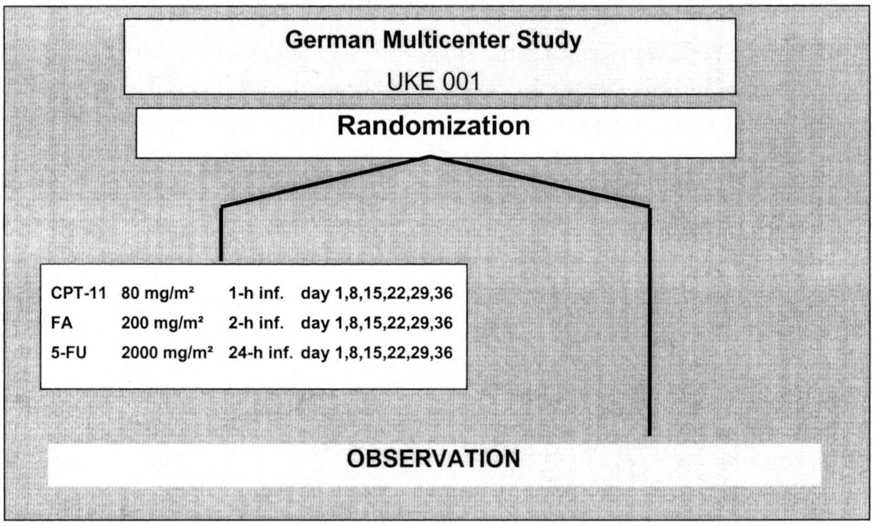

Fig. 3. Design of a German multicenter study on adjuvant chemotherapy after complete resection of hepatic metastases from colorectal carcinomas.

the guidance of Hossfeld and Rogiers (Universitätskrankenhaus Eppendorf, Hamburg, Germany) to compare the effects of weekly doses of CPT-11 + 5-FU/FA to surgery alone (see fig. 3 for study design). The chemotherapeutic agents were administered in 3 cycles of 6 weekly doses, corresponding to a 5-month treatment period. The objective of adjuvant chemotherapy was to achieve a significant reduction in the recurrence rate in the first 2 years after surgery, that is, from approximately 60 to 30%. The preliminary recurrence data from this study should be available around 2003.

Use of Campto plus 5-FU/FA for Neoadjuvant Chemotherapy in Patients with Advanced Colorectal Carcinoma

Neoadjuvant chemotherapy can establish the resectability of formerly inoperable hepatic colorectal metastases. This was demonstrated in a single-center study by Bismuth et al. [2], who found that adjuvant chemotherapy with chronomodulated oxaliplatin plus 5-FU/FA made it possible to completely resect a formerly inoperable tumor in 16% of patients with hepatic colorectal metastases. Of the patients with completely resectable tumors, 54% were alive after 3 years and 40% after 5 years. Hence, their long-term survival rates are similar to those of patients with primary resectability of metastases. These data motivated the EORTC to initiate a corresponding prospective study.

Case reports are available on neoadjuvant polychemotherapy with CPT-11 + 5-FU/FA, but there is a lack of controlled studies. The combination of CPT-11 with 5-FU and FA, administered at weekly intervals, is a very promising strategy, because high response rates of 50–75% occur after only 2 cycles in the majority of patients, corresponding to a treatment period of approximately 3 months [5, 11, 21]. After tumor reduction has been achieved by chemotherapy, local measures can be undertaken for eradication of residual tumor components, especially in the liver, to extend the life expectancy of the patients. Apart from surgery, other local measures include thermoablation with high-frequency electricity or laser technology and cryoablation using liquid nitrogen. In future clinical studies, these measures should be considered and performed whenever possible after the maximum response to chemotherapy has been achieved in the individual patient. This may lead to a new sequence of therapeutic measures to extend the long-term survival.

Summary and Perspectives

Now that two large-scale, randomized studies in patients with metastatic colorectal cancer have shown that combination chemotherapy with CPT-11 plus 5-FU/FA is significantly superior to chemotherapy with 5-FU/FA alone, this combination chemotherapy regimen is now being tested in North America and Europe for adjuvant chemotherapy of stage III colorectal cancer. Considering its proven high antineoplastic activity, this combination of drugs can also be expected to improve long-term survival when used for adjuvant chemotherapy after resection of colorectal metastases due to the more effective killing of residual tumor cells in regionally advanced tumors. The results of these studies will be anxiously awaited in 4 years. Of particular interest is the question of whether high-dose adjuvant chemotherapy with CPT-11 plus 5-FU/FA should be administered when there is only a minimal tumor load or only in the case of tumor recurrence.

Tumor recurrences develop in 50–60% of patients within 2 years of complete resection of liver metastases from colorectal carcinomas. The chances of reducing the rate of recurrence with high-potency chemotherapy appear to be very good. Nonetheless, study UKE 001 will also have to determine whether this chemotherapy regimen is able to increase the long-term survival of patients who are clinically tumor-free. As in patients with stage III colorectal carcinomas, the study should also elucidate the question of whether chemotherapy with CPT-11 + 5-FU/FA is also capable of increasing the long-term survival of patients with inoperable tumor recurrences. Bismuth et al. [2] found that, when used for neoadjuvant chemotherapy, the drug combination established resectability in around 20% of patients with formerly inoperable liver metastases from colorectal carcinomas. This significantly extended the patients' life expectancy. CPT-11 + 5-FU/FA is a highly active drug combination that can achieve high response rates of 50–70%. The maximal response was observed after 3 months of treatment. Hence, neoadjuvant chemotherapy with this drug combination seems to very effectively improve the operability status. Apart from surgical tumor resection, it should also be possible to extend the life expectancy of these patients by less invasive measures, such as thermoablation and cryoablation. Hence, a number of studies will be initiated in the next few years to determine the optimal sequence of therapy measures for colorectal cancer to achieve the maximum extension of the patients' overall life expectancy. Interdisciplinary cooperation between oncologists and surgeons will therefore play a more central role in the treatment of colorectal cancer in the next few years.

References

1 Asahara T, Kikkawa M, Okajima Y, Ojima Y, Toyota K, Nakahara H, Katayama K, Itamoto T, Marubayashi S, One E, Yahata H, Dohi K, Azuma K, Ito K: Studies of postoperative transarterial infusion chemotherapy for liver metastasis of colorectal carcinoma after hepatectomy. Hepatogastroenterology 1998;45:805–811.
2 Bismuth H, Adam R: Reduction of nonresectable liver metastasis from colorectal cancer after oxaliplatin chemotherapy. Semin Oncol 1998;25(suppl 2):40–46.
3 Bradley AL, Chapman WC, Wright JK, Marsh JW, Geevarghese S, Blair KT, Pinson CW: Surgical experience with hepatic colorectal metastasis. Am Surg 1999;65:560–566.
4 Curley S, Roh M, Chase J, Hohn D: Adjuvant hepatic arterial infusion chemotherapy after curative resection of colorectal liver metastases. Am J Surg 1993;166:743–748.
5 Douillard JY, Cunningham D, Roth AD, Germa JR: A randomized phase III trial comparing irinotecan (IRI) + 5-FU/folinic acid (FA) to the same schedule of 5-FU/FA in patients with metastatic colorectal cancer (MCRC) as front line chemotherapy (CT). Proc Am Soc Clin Oncol 1999;18:899 (abstr).
6 Fong Y, Blumgart LH: Hepatic colorectal metastasis: current status of surgical therapy. Oncology (Huntingt) 1998;12:1489–1498.
7 IMPACT: Efficacy of adjuvant fluorouracil and folinic acid in B2 colon cancer. J Clin Oncol 1999; 17:1356–1363.
8 International multicentre pooled analysis of colon cancer trials (IMPACT) investigators: Efficacy of adjuvant fluorouracil and folinic acid in colon cancer. Lancet 1995;345:939–944.
9 Kemeny N, Cohen A, Huang Y, Shi W, Blumgart L, Turnbull A, Sullivan D, Stockman J, Fong Y: Randomized study of hepatic arterial infusion (HAI) and systemic chemotherapy (SYS) versus SYS alone as adjuvant therapy after resection of hepatic metastases from colorectal cancer. Proc Am Soc Clin Oncol1999;18:1011(abstr).
10 Kokudo N, Seki M, Ohta H, Azekura K, Ueno M, Sato T, Moroguchi A, Matsubara T, Takahashi T, Nakajima T, Aiba K: Effects of systemic and regional chemotherapy after hepatic resection for colorectal metastases. Ann Sug Oncol 1998;5:706–712.
11 Lipp R, Hegewisch-Becker S, Popp J, Meyer A, Hossfeld DK: First line treatment of patients with advanced colorectal cancer (CRC) with the combination of CPT-11 and high-dose 5-FU/FA weekly. Deutscher Krebskongress 2000 (abstract).
12 Lorenz M, Müller HH, Schramm H, Gassel HJ, Rau HG, Ridwelski K, Hauss J, Stieger R, Jauch KW, Bechstein WO, Encke A: Randomized trial of surgery versus surgery followed by adjuvant hepatic arterial infusion with 5-fluorouracil and folinic acid for liver metastases of colorectal cancer. German Cooperative on Liver Metastases (Arbeitsgruppe Lebermetastasen). Ann Surg 1998;228: 756–762.
13 Mamounas E, Wieand S, Wolmark N, Bear HD, Atkins JN, Song K, Jones J, Rockette H: Comparative efficacy of adjuvant chemotherapy in patients with Dukes B vs. Dukes C colon cancer: Results from four NSABP adjuvant studies. J Clin Oncol 1999;17:1349–1355.
14 Midgley RS, Kerr DJ: Systemic adjuvant chemotherapy for colorectal cancer; in Bleiber H, Rougiers P, Wilke HJ (eds): Management of Colorectal Cancer. London, Dunitz, 1998, pp 126–137.

15 Moertel CG, Fleming TR, Macdonald JS et al: Fluorouracil plus levamisole as effective adjuvant therapy after resection of stage III colon carcinoma: A final report. Ann Internal Med 1995;122:321–326.
16 Nordic Gastrointestinal Tumour Adjuvant Therapy Group: Expectancy or primary chemotherapy in patients with advanced asymptomatic colorectal cancer: a randomised trial. J Clin Oncol 1992;10: 904–911.
17 Nordlinger B, Giuguet M, Vaillant JC, Balladur P, Boudjema K, Bachellier P, Jaeck D: Surgical resection of colorectal carcinoma metastases to the liver. Cancer 1996;77:1254–1262.
18 O'Connell MJ, Laurie JA, Kahn M, Fitzgibbons RJ Jr, Erlichman C, Shepherd L, Moertel CG, Kocha WI, Pazdur R, Wieand HS, Rubin J, Vukov AM, Donohue JH, Krook JE, Figueredo A: Prospectively randomised trial of postoperative adjuvant chemotherapy in patients with high risk colon cancer. J Clin Oncol 1998;16:295–300.
19 Riesener KP, Winkeltau G, Kasperk R, Cheng L, Schumpelick V: Adjuvant regional arterial port chemotherapy after resection of colorectal liver metastases. Chirurg 1998;69:741–746.
20 Saltz LB, Locker PK, Pirotta N, Elfring GL, Miller LL: Weekly irinotecan (CPT-11), leucovorin (LV) and fluorouracil (FU) is superior to daily x5 LV/FU in patients with previously untreated metastatic colorectal cancer (CRC). Proc Am Soc Clin Oncol 1999;18:898(abstr).
21 Vanhöfer U, Harstrick A, Achterrath W, Lipp R, Maye S, Schöffski P, Köhne CH, Hossfeld DK, Wilke H, Seeber S: Extended phase I study of a weekly schedule of CPT-11, folinic acid and infusional 5-FU as first line chemotherapy (CT) in metastatic colorectal cancer. Onkologie 1999;18: 345.
22 Wolmark N, Rockette H, Fisher B, Wickerham DL, Redmond C, Fisher ER, Jones J, Mamounas EP, Ore L, Petrelli NJ: The benefit of leucovorin-modulated fluorouracil as postoperative adjuvant therapy for primary colon cancer: Results from National Surgical Adjuvant Breast and Bowel Project protocol C-03. J Clin Oncol 1993;11:1879–1887.

ONKOLOGIE

Onkologie 2000;23(suppl 4):23–25

Results with Irinotecan in Gastric Carcinoma

C. H. Köhne S. Casper M. Freund

Abteilung für Hämatologie und Onkologie, Universität Rostock

Introduction

Although the incidence of gastric cancer has continuously decreased over the past few decades, it is still one of the most common malignant diseases worldwide. Moreover, a rapid increase in tumors of the esophagogastric transition has meanwhile been observed [1]. The prognosis of this aggressive tumor is poor, even when detected in the early stages and treated by radical resection [2]. In most cases, metastases are already present at the time of diagnosis. Combination chemotherapy is the treatment of choice for patients with metastatic or locally progressive cancer. Compared to purely supportive treatment, systemic chemotherapy leads to a significant extension of survival and clear improvement in the quality of life with respect to the reduction of tumor-related symptoms. This was demonstrated in various randomized studies [3–5]. However, objective remissions are often only short-term, and most of the patients die of the disease within 1 year. It is therefore necessary to search for new substances with activity in this disease and to incorporate these substances into existing chemotherapeutic regimens. In addition to antimetabolites and anthracyclins, cisplatin is one of the most effective substances for treatment of this disease. The mono-activity of these drugs (objective remission rate) was reported to be 20% [6]. Study findings indicate that continuous infusion of 5-fluorouracil (5-FU) in combination with cisplatin is probably the best reference treatment at present [7]. In randomized studies, investigators have observed remission rates of 40% and median survival times of around 9 months in regimens consisting of 5-FU continuous infusion plus cisplatin in combination with epirubicin (ECF scheme) or mitomycin C (MCF scheme) [8, 9].

Irinotecan (CPT-11) is an S-phase specific semisynthetic derivative of camptothecin that interferes with DNA replication and cell division by inhibiting the enzyme topoisomerase I. The good results with this substance in patients with metastatic colorectal cancer [10] have awakened interest in investigating the efficacy of CPT-11 in gastric cancer.

Mono-Activity of CPT-11 in Gastric Cancer

In 1994, Futatsuki [11] published his findings in 60 patients with metastatic gastric cancer who were treated with 100 mg/m^2 CPT-11 weekly or 150 mg/m^2 CPT-11 biweekly. The objective remission rate of 23% was very promising.

Preliminary data were published by Hecht and co-workers [12]. Weekly therapy with 125 mg/m^2 CPT-11 was administered to 13 patients for 4 consecutive weeks followed by a 2-week break. A complete remission was observed in 1 of the 13 patients. The investigators found that the tolerance of CPT-11 in patients with gastric cancer was lower than expected based on the experiences in patients with colon cancer. However, the cohort of examined patients was rather small for such a conclusion.

In a phase II study performed by 12 European and Israeli centers [13], treatment-naive patients with metastatic gastric carcinomas and measurable tumor disease received CPT-11 at a dose of 350 mg/m^2 for 30 min on day 1; the treatment was repeated every 3 weeks. The primary target variable was the rate of objective remissions, which was evaluated by an independent committee of experts based on assessment of CT images. Secondary target variables were the type of side effects, duration of remissions, and time to tumor progression. All patients received conventional premedication with 5-HT$_3$ antagonists; those with a prior cholinergic syndrome under CPT-11 also received subcutaneous atropine.

A total of 40 patients were admitted to the study; the tumor response was assessable in 35 of them. Complete remission was achieved in 3 patients and partial remission in 4, corresponding to a total remission rate of 20%. The progression-free survival was a median of 2.6 months. The median survival time was 7.5 months; 65, 39 and 20% of the patients were alive after 6, 9 and 12 months, respectively. The most frequent side effect was neutropenia of grade 3 and 4 in 31% of the patients; however, only 1 patient (5%) developed neutropenic fever. The occurrence of 3rd/4th degree diarrhea was observed in 18% of the patients, and 4th degree diarrhea in 8%.

KARGER

Fax +49 761 4 52 07 14
E-mail Information@Karger.de
www.karger.com

Accessible online at:
www.karger.com/journals/onk

PD Dr. med. Claus-Henning Köhne
Abteilung für Hämatologie/Onkologie, Universität Rostock
Ernst-Heydemann-Straße 6, D-18055 Rostock (Germany)
Tel. +49-381-494-7408, Fax -7409
E-mail henning.koehne@med.uni-rostock.de

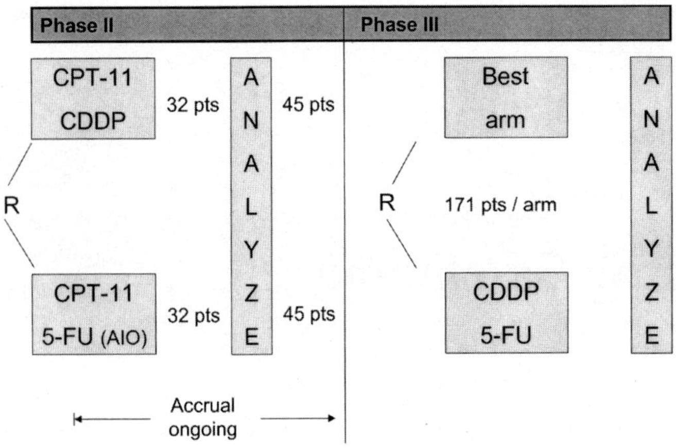

Fig. 1. CPT-11 + cisplatin versus CPT-11 + 5-FU (phase II) and best arm versus cisplatin (CDDP) + 5-FU (phase III).

Severe nausea and vomiting classifiable as grade 3 according to NCI CTC occurred in 1 patient. Alopecia occurred in 45% of the patients, and 48% reported a mild cholinergic syndrome upon direct inquiry. Compared to the mono-activity of other substances, CPT-11 is one of the most effective chemotherapeutic drugs for this tumor entity, especially considering that most of the already established substances have not subjected to such a critical remission analysis. It was also encouraging to find that, in spite of the potential side effects of CPT-11, over 40% the patients reported a subjective improvement of their tumor-related complaints. These findings confirm the Japanese data. The combination of CPT-11 with other active substances therefore appears to be a promising idea.

The feasibility, pharmacokinetic interactions, and possible sequence-dependence of irinotecan and cisplatin were investigated within the scope of a phase I study performed in Rotterdam [14, 15]. Pretreated patients with a maximum of 1 combination chemotherapy or 2 single-agent therapies received irinotecan for 90 min followed by a 3-hour cisplatin infusion on day 1; the cycles were repeated every 3 weeks. The maximum tolerable dose was determined, and the sequence of administration of the two drugs was then reversed. The effect of a prophylactic dose of G-CSF on hematological toxicity was also studied. The investigated irinotecan dose ranged from 175 to 300 mg/m^2, and the cisplatin dose ranged from 60 to 80 mg/m^2. A total of 52 patients were treated within the framework of this study. The dose-limiting toxic side effects were found to be neutropenic fever, diarrhea and fatigue at dose levels of 300 mg/m^2 irinotecan and 80 mg/m^2 cisplatin. The toxicity of the treatment was apparently independent of the sequence of administration of the cytostatic agents. The recommended doses for phase II studies were 260 mg/m^2 irinotecan plus 80 mg/m^2 cisplatin every 2 weeks for chemotherapy-naive patients. The authors recommend that the irinotecan dose be reduced to 200 mg/m^2 in pretreated patients or those with poor general health. The pharmacokinetic studies showed no interactions between the two substances. The inverted order of the administration also had no effect on the pharmacokinetics of CPT-11.

Boku et al. [16] treated 44 patients with a 90-min infusion of 70 mg/m^2 irinotecan on days 1 and 15 in combination with a 2-hour infusion of 80 mg/m^2 cisplatin on day 1. The therapy was repeated every 4–6 weeks. An objective remission was observed in 59% of a total of 29 non-pretreated patients (95%, CI 39–77%). 15 patients had received prior chemotherapeutic treatment; an objective remission was observed in 27% of them (95%, CI 8–55%).

Shirao and co-workers [17] treated 24 patients with the same CPT-11 and cisplatin dosage schedule used by Boku's team. Neutropenia was the dose-limiting factor. An objective remission was observed in 7 of 20 pretreated patients and in 3 of 4 non-pretreated patients. The overall remission rate for all 24 patients was 42% (95%, CI 22–61%). The median survival time in the treatment-naive patients was 323 days, and that for the total group of 24 patients studied was 272 days. The most frequent side effect was neutropenia with grade 4 in 57% of the patients; 21% of the patients had diarrhea grades 3 or 4 [16].

Weekly cisplatin and CPT-11 administration was investigated at the Memorial Sloan Kettering Cancer Center (MSKCC) and at the M.D. Anderson Cancer Center (MDACC). The cisplatin dose was 30 mg/m^2 in combination with 65 mg/m^2 of CPT-11. Therapy was repeated at weekly intervals. Ilson et al. [18] achieved a response rate of 18% in 14 patients, some of whom had already been pretreated. Ajani and co-workers [19] treated 35 patients, 8 of which had already been pretreated. The remission rate for the non-pretreated patients was 51%. Four of the 8 pretreated patients (50%) responded to this form of combination therapy. Treatment delays were necessary in 9% of the total of 308 cycles. 17 of the 35 patients additionally received G-CSF, and 9 of the 35 patients had to be hospitalized because of side effects. These findings imply that combination chemotherapy with CPT-11 is a very effective regimen in patients with gastric cancer, and that it should be evaluated in further systematic clinical trials.

Ongoing Investigations

Apart from cisplatin, continuous 5-FU infusion is one of the most important pillars of systemic chemotherapy of gastric cancer. The combination of continuous 5-FU infusions with CPT-11 therefore seems to suggest itself. A number of interesting findings on the use of this type of combination chemotherapy in patients with metastatic colorectal carcinoma cancer have already been published [20]. The tolerance of the AIO scheme in combination with CPT-11 and of the De Gramont scheme in combination with CPT-11 is sufficiently known [21]. It would therefore appear wise to test the efficacy of the combination in gastric cancer. Therefore, investigators are currently comparing the activity of the AIO scheme in combination with CPT-11 to therapy with CPT-11 plus cisplatin within the framework of a randomized phase II study. Using a pick-the-winner design, the most promising combination will be selected after 45 patients have been recruited to each treatment arm. The selected combination therapy will then be continued in a phase III study and compared to reference therapy with continuous 5-FU infusion plus cisplatin (fig. 1). This study will supply important findings regarding the value of CPT-11 in gastric cancer. For now, the use of CPT-11 in patients with gastric cancer should preferably be limited to the framework of clinical studies. Compared to patients with metastatic colorectal cancer, patients with gastric cancer are more often in a worse state of general health and more frequently experience tumor-related symptoms, such as lack of appetite and weight loss. Therefore, they may also have a poorer tolerance to chemotherapy. Careful selection of the patients and the use of intensive supportive care measures combined with the increasing body of findings on CPT-11 should help to make this type of therapy a safe alternative for patients with gastric cancer.

References

1 Blot WJ, Devesa,SS, Kneller RW, Fraumeni JF Jr.: Rising incidence of adenocarcinoma of the esophagus and gastric cardia [see comments]. JAMA 1991;265:1287–1289.

2 Hendlisz A, Bleiberg H: Diagnosis and treatment of gastric cancer. Drugs 1995;49:711–720.

3 Murad AM, Santiago FF, Petroianu A, Rocha PR, Rodrigues MA, Rausch M: Modified therapy with 5-fluorouracil, doxorubicin, and methotrexate in advanced gastric cancer. Cancer 1993;72:37–41.

4 Pyrhönen S, Kouri M: Epirubicin-sequential methotrexate-5-FU (EMF) in the treatment of colorectal cancer. Proc Am Soc Clin Oncol 1991; 10:442.

5 Glimelius B, Ekstrom K, Hoffman K, Graf W, Sjoden PO, Haglund U, Svensson C, Enander LK, Linne T, Sellstrom H, Heuman R: Randomized comparison between chemotherapy plus best supportive care with best supportive care in advanced gastric cancer. Ann Oncol 1997;8:163–168.

6 Alexander HR, Kelsen D, Tepper J: Cancer of the stomach. Cancer 1997;5:1012–1054.

7 Wilke H, Vanhöfer U, Fink U, Köhne-Wömpner CH, Stahl M, Klaassen U, Strumberg D, Eberhardt W, Schmoll HJ, Achterrath W, Seeber S: Weekly high-dose FU/folinic acid plus biweekly cisplatin = group A or HD-FU/FA plus alternating cisplatin/ epidoxorubicin = group B for gastric cancer. esmo 1994;19:P397.

8 Webb A, Cunningham D, Scarffe JH, Harper P, Norman A, Joffe JK, Hughes M, Mansi J, Findlay M, Hill A, Oates J, Nicolson M, Hickish T, O'Brien M, Iveson T, Watson M, Underhill C, Wardley A, Meehan M: Randomized trial comparing epirubicin, cisplatin, and fluorouracil versus fluorouracil, doxorubicin, and methotrexate in advanced esophagogastric cancer. J Clin Oncol 1997;15:261–267.

9 Ross PJ, Cunningham D, Scarffe JH, Nicolson M, Seymour M, Harper P, Price T, Hill A, Anderson H, Iveson T, Hickish T, Lofts F, Norman A: Results of a randomized trial comparing ECF with MCF in advanced esophago-gastric cancer. Proc Am Soc Clin Oncol 1999;18:272a.

10 Rougier P, Van CE, Bajetta E, Niederle N, Possinger K, Labianca R, Navarro M, Morant R, Bleiberg H, Wils J, Awad L, Herait P, Jacques C: Randomised trial of irinotecan versus fluorouracil by continuous infusion after fluorouracil failure in patients with metastatic colorectal cancer [published erratum appears in Lancet 1998 Nov 14; 352(9140):1634]. Lancet 1998;352:1407– 1412.

11 Futatsuki K, Wakui A, Nakao I, Sakata Y, Kambe M, Shimada Y, Yoshino M, Taguchi T, Ogawa N: [Late phase II study of irinotecan hydrochloride (CPT-11) in advanced gastric cancer. CPT-11 Gastrointestinal Cancer Study Group]. Gan To Kagaku Ryoho 1994;21:1033–1038.

12 Hecht JR, Parson M, Rosen L: A phase II trial of irinotecan (CPT-11) in patients with adenocarcinoma of the esophagus and gastric cardia. Proc Am Soc Clin Oncol 1999;18:278a.

13 Köhne CH, Thuss-Patience P, Catane R: Final results of a phase II trial of CPT-11 in patients with advanced gastric cancer. Proc Am Soc Clin Oncol 1999;18:258.

14 de Jonge MJ, Sparreboom A, Planting AS, Der Burg ME, Boer-Dennert MM, Steeg J, Jacques C, Verweij J: Phase I study of 3-week schedule of irinotecan combined with cisplatin in patients with advanced solid tumors. J Clin Oncol 2000;18:187.

15 de Jonge MJ, Verweij J, de Bruijn J, Prouwer E, Mathijssen RH, van Alphen RJ, Boer-Dennert MM, Vernillet L, Jacques C, Sparreboom A: Pharmacokinetic, metabolic, and pharmacodynamic profiles in a dose-escalating study of irinotecan and cisplatin. J Clin Oncol 2000;18:195.

16 Boku N, Ohtsu A, Shimada Y, Shirao K, Seki S, Saito H, Sakata Y, Hyodo I: Phase II study of a combination of irinotecan and cisplatin against metastatic gastric cancer. J Clin Oncol 1999;17: 319–323.

17 Shirao K, Shimada Y, Kondo H, Saito D, Yamao T, Ono H, Yokoyama T, Fukuda H, Oka M, Watanabe Y, Ohtsu A, Boku N, Fujii T, Oda Y, Muro K, Yoshida, S: Phase I-II study of irinotecan hydrochloride combined with cisplatin in patients with advanced gastric cancer. J Clin Oncol 1997;15: 921–927.

18 Ilson D, Enzinger PC, Saltz L, O'Reilly EM, Schwartz G, Sharma SK, Gollub M: Phase II trial of weekly irinotecan + cisplatin in advanced gastric cancer. Proc Am Soc Clin Oncol 1999;18:994.

19 Ajani J, Fairweather J, Pisters PW, Feig B, Hargraves K: Phase II study of CPT-11 plus cisplatin in patients with advanced gastric and GE junction carcinomas. Proc Am Soc Clin Oncol 1999;18:245a.

20 Vanhoefer U, Harstrick A, Köhne CH, Achterrath W, Rustum YM, Seeber S, Wilke H: Phase I study of a weekly schedule of irinotecan, high-dose leucovorin, and infusional fluorouracil as first-line chemotherapy in patients with advanced colorectal cancer. J Clin Oncol 1999;17:907–913.

21 Douillard JY, Cunningham D, Roth A, Germa JR, James RD, Karasek P, Jandik T, Iveson T, Carmichael J, Gruia G, Dembak M, Sibaud D, Rougier P: A randomized phase III trial comparing irinotecan (IRI) + 5-FU/folinic acid (FA) to the same schedule of 5-FU/FA in patients (pts) with metastatic colorectal cancer (MCRC) as front line chemotherapy (CT). Proc Am Soc Clin Oncol 1999;18:233a.

ONKOLOGIE

Onkologie 2000;23(suppl 4):26–28

Irinotecan in Esophageal Cancer: First Results

P. Reichardt

Medizinische Klinik m. S. Hämatologie, Onkologie und Tumorimmunologie, Robert-Rössle-Klinik, Universitätsklinikum Charité

Key Words
Esophageal cancer · Chemotherapy · Irinotecan

Summary
Esophageal cancer is a major health problem, being among the 10 most frequent cancers in the world. The prognosis is very poor with 5-year survival rates below 10% due to local recurrent or metastatic disease. Treatment strategies consist of operative procedures, radiotherapy and chemotherapy. There is strong and increasing evidence in favor of multimodality approaches, both in potentially resectable and locally advanced disease. While single-modality neoadjuvant or adjuvant radiation and chemotherapy do not improve survival rates compared to surgery alone, the combination of chemotherapy with radiotherapy is significantly superior to radiotherapy alone. For multimodality treatment, the combination of cisplatinum and infusional 5-fluorouracil is considered standard of care. For patients with metastatic disease, single-agent chemotherapy, preferably on an outpatient basis, is the treatment of choice. In the search for new active agents against cancer of the esophagus and the gastroesophageal junction, evaluation of irinotecan (CPT-11, Campto®) as a single agent, in combination with cisplatinum, or in conjunction with radiation therapy has been started with promising first results.

Schlüsselwörter
Ösophaguskarzinom · Chemotherapie · Irinotecan

Zusammenfassung
Das Ösophaguskarzinom gehört zu den zehn häufigsten Krebsarten weltweit. Die 5-Jahres-Überlebensrate liegt unter 10%. Hauptprobleme sind sowohl Lokalrezidive als auch Fernmetastasen. Die Behandlungsoptionen bestehen aus Operation, Bestrahlung und Chemotherapie, wobei multimodalen Therapiekonzepten aufgrund ihrer wahrscheinlichen Überlegenheit zunehmende Bedeutung zukommt. Bestrahlung oder Chemotherapie als alleinige adjuvante Therapien verbessern die Ergebnisse der Chirurgie nicht. Die kombinierte Radiochemotherapie hat sich indessen einer alleinigen Bestrahlung als eindeutig überlegen erwiesen. Für den Einsatz im Rahmen einer multimodaler Therapie stellt die Kombination von Cisplatin und 5-Fluorouracil-Dauerinfusion die Chemotherapie der Wahl dar. Patienten mit metastasierendem Ösophaguskarzinom sollten vorzugsweise eine ambulant durchführbare Monotherapie erhalten. Auf der Suche nach neuen aktiven Substanzen wurden mit Irinotecan (CPT-11, Campto®) in der Monotherapie, in Kombination mit Cisplatin oder gemeinsam mit einer Strahlentherapie erste Erfolge gesehen.

Introduction

Esophageal cancer is a major health problem, being among the 10 most frequent cancers in the world. The incidence varies from very high numbers in endemic regions to around 4 out of 100.000 in the western world. Patients are predominantly males around 65 years of age. Among other risk factors, alcohol consumption and smoking play a major role. The predominant histologic subtype is squamous cell cancer, accounting for approximately 60–70% of cases. Adenocarcinomas are seen in about 30–40% of patients, predominantly in the gastroesophageal junction. The incidence of adenocarcinomas has been increasing rapidly over the last years, the reasons still being unknown.

KARGER

Fax +49 761 4 52 07 14
E-mail Information@Karger.de
www.karger.com

Accessible online at:
www.karger.com/journals/onk

Dr. med. Peter Reichardt
Medizinische Klinik m. S. Hämatologie, Onkologie und Tumorimmunologie
Robert-Rössle-Klinik, Universitätsklinikum Charité
D-13122 Berlin (Germany)
Tel. 030-941712-10, Fax -19
E-mail reichardt@rrk-berlin.de

The prognosis is generally very poor with 5-year survival rates clearly below 10%. Only patients with small, potentially resectable tumors have a somewhat better prognosis with survival rates of about 20%.

Treatment strategies consist of operative procedures, radiotherapy and chemotherapy. There is strong and increasing evidence in favor of multimodality approaches, both in potentially resectable and locally advanced disease. Chemotherapy is intended for shrinkage of the local tumor, leading to improved resection rates, and to control systemic spread with improvement of survival.

While single-modality neoadjuvant or adjuvant radiation [1, 2] and chemotherapy [3, 4] do not improve survival rates compared to surgery alone, the combination of chemotherapy with radiotherapy is significantly superior to radiotherapy alone [5]. Two randomized studies showed an improved disease-free or even overall survival for preoperative chemoradiation followed by surgery versus surgery alone [6, 7]. Further evidence from nonrandomized or retrospective trials clearly supports the finding that a complete response to neoadjuvant chemoradiation therapy is associated with prolonged survival [8, 9]. Therefore, to improve overall outcome, more effective preoperative treatment is required, using complete remission as a surrogate marker.

Chemotherapy of Esophageal Cancer

Esophageal cancer, both squamous cell and adenocarcinoma, is modestly chemosensitive. Single-agent activity has been reported for only few drugs including bleomycin, 5-fluorouracil (5-FU), mitomycin C, doxorubicin, methotrexate, cisplatinum, vinorelbine, and paclitaxel. Combination chemotherapy results in slightly higher response rates in a range of 30–40%. However, responses are mostly partial and of rather short duration, so that combination chemotherapy should only be considered for neoadjuvant treatment as part of a multimodality approach. The combination of cisplatinum and infusional 5-FU is considered standard of care for this indication [4, 5]. Patients with metastatic disease are mostly candidates for single-agent chemotherapy, preferably on an outpatient basis. Possible exceptions are younger patients with good performance status. In the case of recurrence after cisplatinum-based combination chemotherapy, further chemotherapy can not be recommended on a routine basis. Some activity has been reported for paclitaxel and docetaxel [10], but second-line treatment should be restricted to patients with good performance status and only be used within controlled clinical trials.

Since the intensification of currently used chemotherapy regimens is highly limited by its toxicity, future research should be focused on the identification of new active drugs to be used either as single agents or as part of combination chemotherapy.

Irinotecan in Esophageal Cancer

Irinotecan, a semisynthetic derivative of camptothecine, acting by inhibition of the enzyme topoisomerase I, has shown significant activity against gastrointestinal adenocarcinomas of the colorectum and the stomach. Based on these data, irinotecan has been evaluated in esophageal and gastroesophageal junction cancers as a single agent, in combination with cisplatinum or in conjunction with radiation therapy.

Enzinger et al. [11] from Memorial Sloan-Kettering Cancer Center have reported on a phase II trial of cisplatinum and irinotecan in patients with advanced esophageal cancer. Both drugs were given weekly at a dose of 30 and 65 mg/m^2, respectively, times four with a 2-week break. 21 previously untreated patients with adenocarcinoma or squamous cell carcinoma were entered in this study. The toxicity was rather mild with 34% grade 3 or 4 neutropenia and 21% grade 2 or 3 diarrhea. Responses were seen in 6 out of 11 evaluable patients with adenocarcinoma and 3 out of 6 patients with squamous cell cancer. Minor responses occurred in another 5 of 17 patients. The authors conclude that this combination should be tested against other cisplatinum-containing regimens. Further data on the combination of weekly cisplatinum and irinotecan were published by Ajani et al. [12] from M. D. Anderson Cancer Center. 35 patients with advanced gastric or gastroesophageal junction carcinomas, the majority being previously untreated, received a median number of 3 cycles. The doses used were 30 and 65 mg/m^2, respectively. In pretreated patients, irinotecan was reduced to 50 mg/m^2 per week. Toxicity consisted of neutropenia and diarrhea, leading to a delay of weekly doses in 9% and a cancellation in 7%. 26% of patients had to be hospitalized at least once for toxicity management. 13 out of 25 evaluable patients, who were previously untreated, achieved a partial (10) or complete (3) response. Comparable results were seen in 8 evaluable pretreated patients with 4 of them responding to the treatment.

The single-agent activity of irinotecan in patients with adenocarcinomas of the esophagus and gastric cardia has been evaluated by Hecht et al. [13] from the University of California, Los Angeles. 13 patients, most of them pretreated, were given a standard weekly regimen using 125 mg/m^2 times four with a 2-week rest. In 7 out of 13 patients who received more than 1 cycle, 1 complete remission, lasting for more than 24 weeks, and 5 disease stabilizations for 12 to more than 36 weeks were seen, suggesting some activity of this treatment regimen even in pretreated patients. Grade 3 diarrhea and neutropenia occurred in 57 and 42% of patients, respectively.

The radiosensitizing properties of irinotecan in patients with locally advanced upper gastrointestinal carcinomas are studied by Fairweather et al. [14] from the M. D. Anderson Cancer Center. So far, 11 patients, 3 of them after pretreatment with platinum-based chemotherapy, have been treated in a phase I study using increasing doses of irinotecan weekly in combination with 45 Gy of external-beam radiation over 5 weeks. The currently used dose of irinotecan is reported to be 50 mg/m^2. Dose escalation is ongoing until maximum tolerated dose (MTD), which has not been reached yet. Apart from 1 lethal hemorrhage from the cancer in the 4th week of treatment, no other major toxicity was noted. The authors state that radiologic and endoscopic responses have been observed.

Few patients with esophageal cancer have been included in irinotecan-based combination chemotherapy trials with oxaliplatin and raltitrexet. However, the numbers are too small to draw any conclusions.

Conclusions

Early reports on mostly ongoing trials indicate activity of irinotecan alone or in combination with cisplatinum or radiotherapy against cancers of the esophagus and the gastroesophageal junction.

Future trials should focus on single-agent activity of irinotecan in previously untreated patients with advanced or metastatic esophageal cancer. In operable or locally advanced disease, irinotecan should be studied as part of a combination chemotherapy in the context of a multimodality approach.

References

1 Teniere P, Hay JM, Fingerhut A, Fagniez PL: Postoperative radiation therapy does not increase survival after curative resection for squamous cell carcinoma of the middle and lower esophagus as shown by a multicenter controlled trial. Surg Gynecol Obstet 1991;173:123–130.

2 Schlag P: Randomized trial of preoperative chemotherapy for squamous cell cancer of the esophagus. Arch Surg 1992;127:1446–1450.

3 Kelsen DP, Ginsberg R, Pajak TF, Sheahan DG, Gunderson L, Mortimer J, Estes N, Haller DG, Ajani J, Kocha W, Minsky BD, Roth JA: Chemotherapy followed by surgery compared with surgery alone for localized esophageal cancer. N Engl J Med 1998;339:1979–1984.

4 Herskovic A, Martz K, al Sarraf M, Leichmann L, Brindle J, Vaitkevicius V, Cooper J, Byhardt R, Davis L, Emami B: Combined chemotherapy and radiotherapy compared with radiotherapy alone in patients with cancer of the esophagus. N Engl J Med 1992;326:1593–1598.

5 Gignoux M, Roussel A, Paillot B, Gillet M, Schlag P, Favre JP, Dalesio O, Buyse M, Duez N: The value of preoperative radiotherapy in esophageal cancer: Results of a study of the EORTC. World J Surg 1981;11:426–432.

6 Walsh TN, Noonan N, Hollywood D, Kelly A, Keeling N, Hennessy TP: A comparison of multimodal therapy and surgery for esophageal adenocarcinoma. N Engl J Med 1996;335:462–467.

7 Bosset JF, Gignoux M, Triboulet JP, Tiret E, Mantion G, Elias D, Lozach P, Ollier JC, Pavy JJ, Mercier M, Sahmoud T: Chemoradiotherapy followed by surgery compared with surgery alone in squamous cell cancer of the esophagus. N Engl J Med 1997; 337:161–167.

8 Bates BA, Detterbeck FC, Bernard SA, Qaqish BF, Tepper JE: Concurrent radiation therapy and chemotherapy followed by esophagectomy for localized esophageal carcinoma. J Clin Oncol 1996;14: 156–163.

9 Carey RW, Hilgenberg AD, Wilkins EW Jr, Choi NC, Mathisen DJ, Grillo HC, Wain JC, Logan DL, Bromberg C: Long-term follow-up of neoadjuvant chemotherapy with 5-fluorouracil and cisplatin with surgical resection and possible postoperative radiotherapy and/or chemotherapy in squamous cell carcinoma of the esophagus. Cancer Invest 1993;11:99–105.

10 Fenchel K, Karthaus M, Steffens C, Dreher K, Boehme V, Pralle H, Kubicka S, Weber C, Stoffregen C: Taxanes: An effective 2nd line treatment of advanced esophageal cancer – A randomized trial. Proc Am Soc Clin Oncol 1999;18:283a.

11 Enzinger PC, Ilson DH, Saltz LB, O'Reilly EM, Gotlub MJ, DeGroff JA, Kelsen DP: A phase II trial of cisplatin and irinotecan in patients with advanced esophageal cancer. Proc Am Soc Clin Oncol 1998;17:282a.

12 Ajani JA, Fairweather J, Pisters PW, Feig BW, Hargraves K, Ghamsanngavej C: Phase II study of CPT-11 plus cisplatin in patients with advanced gastric and GE junction carcinomas. Proc Am Soc Clin Oncol 1999;18:241a.

13 Hecht JR, Parson M, Rosen LS: A phase II trial of irinotecan (CPT-11) in patients with adenocarcinoma of the esophagus and gastric cardia. Proc Am Soc Clin Oncol 1999;18:287a.

14 Fairweather J, Ajani JA, Komaki R, Janjan NA, Pisters PW, Mansfield PF, Walsh GL, Delcios ME, Lynch PM, Raijman I, Feig BW, Hargraves K: Phase I study of CPT-11 plus radiotherapy in patients with locally advanced upper GI carcinomas. Proc Am Soc Clin Oncol 1999;18:283a.

ONKOLOGIE

Onkologie 2000;23(suppl 4):29–30

Are Biliary Tract and Gallbladder Carcinomas Treatable with Irinotecan?

H. Oettle H. Riess

Medizinische Klinik und Poliklinik m.S. Hämatologie und Onkologie, Medizinische Fakultät der Humboldt Universität zu Berlin

Introduction

Biliary carcinomas, especially those of the gallbladder, are the 7th most common form of cancer in women and the 10th most common form in men. Carcinomas of the extrahepatic bile ducts are rare. These tumors are mainly found in the elderly with a peak incidence between the ages of 60 and 80 years. The presence of gallstones can promote the development of biliary carcinomas. The risk of cancer is approximately 10 times higher in patients with asymptomatic gallstones larger than 3 cm in diameter. There is a risk of 20–60% in patients with a so-called porcelain gallbladder (intramural calcification). The incidence of gallbladder cancer is also increased in patients with gallbladder polyps. Therefore, surgical resection is also indicated in patients with polyps larger than 0.5 cm in diameter. There is also an increased risk associated with the chronic reflux of pancreatic juice in patients with pancreaticobiliary ductal anomalies. 80% of all gallbladder carcinomas are located in the fundus and corpus regions. Tumors in these regions can lead to early infiltration per continuitatem and to hematogenic spreading of the tumor into the liver. Tumors in the region of the hepatic bifurcation (Klatskin's tumors) exhibit slower growth. Even when these tumors are large, lymphogenous spread occurs relatively late and mainly involves the regional portal lymph nodes. Hematogenic spread of gallbladder carcinomas occurs mainly via the gallbladder veins with direct intrahepatic connections to the branches of the portal vein. This is difficult to distinguish from local infiltration. Peritoneal metastases are present in around 20% of cases at the time of diagnosis. Additional hematogenic spreading occurs mainly in the lungs and the bone (pulmonary metastases in 10–20% of cases). Hematogenic spreading to the adrenal gland, skin, ovaries, and spleen may also occur.

The different tumor types – adenocarcinoma (80%), undifferentiated carcinoma (10%), papillary adenocarcinoma (5%), and mucinous adenocarcinoma (5%) – occur in all parts of the biliary tract. The papillary adenocarcinoma is especially common in the ampullar region and has the best prognosis of all carcinomas. Carcinoids, malignant melanomas, and sarcomas are very rare malignant tumors in the region of the efferent bile ducts.

The symptoms are usually unspecific: right epigastric complaints (75%), nausea and vomiting (30%), and weight loss (30%) are common. Jaundice occurs in around 40% of cases, usually in those with advanced tumor invasion. Laboratory tests may reveal elevated levels of tumor markers CA 19-9 and/or CEA. Ultrasound, abdominal computed tomography, endoscopic retrograde cholangiopancreatography (ERCP), and percutaneous transhepatic cholangiography are used for diagnostic imaging. In patients with small primary tumors located near the serosa, gallbladder resection may suffice for curative tumor therapy. If the tumor is located in the gallbladder bed of the liver or is a T2/T3 tumor, atypical hepatectomy of the gallbladder bed must also be performed. The percentage of potentially resectable carcinomas of the gallbladder is only around 15–30%. The 5-year survival rate after potentially curative resection is reported to be 10–60% for carcinomas of the gallbladder. Neither radiotherapy nor chemotherapy has a curative therapy potential.

There is no standard chemotherapy regimen for advanced tumors of the biliary tract and gallbladder. Mitomycin C (MMC) and 5-fluorouracil (5-FU) are the most extensively studied single agents for systemic treatment of biliary tract cancer. Despite early reports that the single agent MMC achieved an encouraging response rate of 47% in 15 patients with biliary cancer, these results could not be confirmed in later studies [1].

As tumors of the biliary tree progress by local spreading rather than by distant metastasis, a regional chemotherapeutic strategy would appear to be a logical approach. Arterial intra-

KARGER

Fax +49 761 4 52 07 14
E-mail Information@Karger.de
www.karger.com

Accessible online at:
www.karger.com/journals/onk

Dr. H. Oettle
Charité Campus Virchow Klinikum
Medizinische Klinik und Poliklinik m.S. Hämatologie und Onkologie
Augustenburger Platz 1, D-13353 Berlin (Germany)
Tel. 0049 30 45053-222; Fax -959
E-mail helmut.oettle@charite.de

hepatic infusion of chemotherapeutic agents has achieved promising results in the treatment of hepatic metastases from colorectal cancer. The anatomical situation is an additional advantage. The lower bile duct branches are mainly supplied by the gastroduodenal and superior mesenteric arteries, whereas the upper biliary tree and gallbladder are mainly supplied by the hepatic artery.

Because of its high hepatic extraction rate and proven activity, floxuridine (FUdR) is the most thoroughly evaluated agent for treatment of colorectal and advanced biliary tract cancer. Despite the elegant underlying biochemical rationale, the only data available at the moment is on intrahepatic infusion of the cytotoxic agents. Some studies have yielded promising results with response rates of up to 78% (albeit only in relatively small groups of patients). Nonetheless, it is still too soon to determine whether this form of treatment has any advantages over systemic chemotherapy.

Apart from the well-known and widely used antineoplastic drugs, newer agents have also been tested for their efficacy in the treatment of biliary cancer. Gemcitabine prevailed over 5-FU as the standard drug for treatment of advanced pancreatic cancer since it is superior with respect to tumor-related symptoms and response rate. Considering the histogenetic relationship between the pancreas and the bile ducts, a therapeutic approach also appears to be prudent in this case. Weismann et al. [2] reported on 8 cases of inoperable cholangiocarcinoma treated with gemcitabine. A dose of 1200 mg/m^2 was administered into hepatic artery as a 30-min infusion via an intra-arterial catheter on 2 consecutive days. The treatment cycles were repeated at 4-week intervals. The median number of cycles was 2 (range 1–6). Repeated insertion of the intra-arterial catheter was possible in all patients requiring repeated treatment. The treatment resulted in 1 complete remission (12.5%), 1 partial remission (12.5%), and 3 stabilizations (37.5%) of cholangiocarcinoma. The median survival cannot yet be determined after only 11 months of observation.

Interestingly enough, there is only very little data available on CPT-11 (irinotecan, Campto®) although it would appear to be a very interesting antineoplastic agent for this tumor entity due to its metabolic profile. Irinotecan, a semisynthetic derivative of camptothecin, is a potent inhibitor of topoisomerase I [3–4]. Within the body, irinotecan is converted to a more active metabolite (SN-38), mainly in the liver. Murine studies suggest that the liver may concentrate irinotecan, convert it to SN-38, and eliminate both compounds via biliary excretion. The plasma concentrations can be determined using 2- or 3-compartment models; the mean terminal half-lives range from 5 to 27 hours. 65% of irinotecan is bound to plasma proteins compared to 95% of SN-38. Maximum concentrations of SN-38 are reached about 1 hour after the beginning of a short intravenous infusion. Irinotecan is extensively metabolized in the liver. The cumulative biliary excretion of irinotecan is 25% compared to 2% for SN-38 glucuronide and about 1% for SN-38. Only small fractions of irinotecan and its metabolites are eliminated in the urine. Larger fractions are eliminated in the bile, and there is an enterohepatic cycle of SN-38 glucuronide and SN-38. The later metabolism of SN-38 to a beta-glucuronide conjugate represents a major pathway of detoxification and plays an important role in determining the toxicity of irinotecan in a clinical setting. The main dose-limiting toxic effect of irinotecan is diarrhea, which occurs 7–10 days after treatment and can be life-threatening when associated with neutropenia, another frequent side effect. Stuart et al. [5] published the results of a small-scale study in 8 patients with adenocarcinomas of the efferent biliary tract. A partial remission has been observed to date. Single case reports suggest that irinotecan has antitumor activity. Phase II studies are warranted.

Considering the aforementioned facts, the combination of gemcitabine plus irinotecan appears to be a promising new treatment option and is a favored study concept. On the whole, the results of single-agent chemotherapy have been disappointing, and most of the drugs studied have been rather ineffective in terms of inducing an objective response to treatment. Since no data on the effects of single-agent therapy on survival and quality of life compared to untreated patients have yet been published, none of the single-agent chemotherapy regimens studied so far can be recommended for routine clinical use. Various combination chemotherapy regimens have been tested for treatment of advanced biliary cancer in phase II studies, but response rates of more than 30% have been difficult to achieve.

References

1 Taal BG, Audisio RA, Bleiberg H, Blijham GH, Neijt JP, Veenhof CH, Duez N, Sahmoud T: Phase II trial of mitomycin C (MMC) in advanced gallbladder and biliary tree carcinoma. An EORTC Gastrointestinal Tract Cancer Cooperative Group Study. Ann Oncol 1993;4:607–609.

2 Weisman A, Ludwig H: Intraarterial Gemcitabine for treatment of inoperable pancreatic and cholangio-arcinoma. Proc Am Soc Clin Oncol 1999, abstr 1170.

3 Chabot GG: Clinical pharmacokinetics of irinotecan. Clin Pharmacokinet 1997; 33:245–259.

4 Robert J, Rivory L: Pharmacology of irinotecan. Drugs Today 1998;34:777–803.

5 Stuart KE, Sanz-Altamira PM, Raeburn L, O'Reilly E, Steger C, Semple D, Kemeny N, Ilson D, Kelsen D, Saltz L: A phase II trial of irinotecan (CPT-11) for biliary tree carcinoma. Proc Am Soc Clin Oncol 1998;abstr 1167.

ONKOLOGIE

Onkologie 2000;23(suppl 4):31–33

Irinotecan in Radiation Oncology

G. Klautke R. Fietkau

Klinik und Poliklinik für Strahlentherapie, Universität Rostock

Introduction

Radiotherapy is the best treatment modality to achieve long-term local control of solid tumors, considered as inoperable by the surgeon. The objective of concurrent radiochemotherapy is to achieve better local control by means of additive or synergistic effects of radiotherapy and the antineoplastic drug. Moreover, preoperative radiochemotherapy may lead to a significant downstaging of the tumor, permitting radical surgery with a curative intent. Another target of simultaneous radiochemotherapy is the reduction of distant metastases using the systemic effects of chemotherapy.

The combined toxicity of radiation and chemotherapy must be balanced in that way, that both the radiotherapy and the antineoplastic drug can be administered in a sufficient high dosage. Dose compromises must be avoided.

This review summarizes the experiences with irinotecan, an antineoplastic agent inhibiting the eukaryotic DNA topoisomerase I, combined with concurrent radiotherapy.

Rationale for the Combination of Radiation and Irinotecan

Irinotecan, a water-soluble semisynthetic derivative of camptothecin, is an antineoplastic agent, inhibiting the eukaryotic DNA topoisomerase I by interaction between the stabilized cleavage complex and the advancing replication machinery. The resulting collision provokes an arrest of the progression fork and irreversible DNA strand break [1, 2]. These damages can finally lead to cell death. Cancer tissues with high topoisomerase I levels are very sensitive to irinotecan [2–5]. Damages of DNA by radiation are often repaired by DNA repair systems. Therefore, the inhibition of DNA repair by irinotecan leads to an increased efficacy of irradiation. This radiation sensitization effect was shown in numerous cell culture experiments [6–10]. In this context, it is very interesting that the topoisomerase I enzyme works without ATP, and therefore, also in hypoxic tissue. So radiosensitizing by irinotecan is also possible in hypoxic tumor regions [7].

Beside the synergistic effect of radiation and the antineoplastic drug, the other important precondition of concurrent radiochemotherapy is, that the applied drug has demonstrated single-agent activity against the tumor treated. Phase I and II trials have proven a significant activity of irinotecan in patients with glioblastoma, esophageal, gastric and pancreatic cancer, small-cell (SCLC) and non-small-cell lung cancer (NSCLC), squamous cell cancer of the cervix, and especially colon and rectal cancer [11–28].

Phase I/II Trials of Concurrent Radiochemotherapy with Irinotecan

There are only few reports concerning concomitant radiochemotherapy with irinotecan. Data exist for head and neck cancer, NSCLC, and rectal cancer (table 1).

Koukourakis et al. [29] recruited 12 patients with locally advanced head and neck cancer to a dose escalation protocol with docetaxel (20, 20, 25 mg/m^2) and irinotecan (25, 40, 55 mg/m^2) weekly concurrently with a conventionally fractionated radiotherapy (2 Gy/day, 5 days/week) to a total dose of 66–70 Gy. There was no hematological toxicity grade 3 or 4 , and 5 patients had a mucositis grade 3 or 4. The observed response rate was 100% (9/12 complete response (CR), 3/12 partial response (PR)).

The studies of irinotecan and concurrent radiation in patients with locally advanced NSCLC stage III A/B can be divided into two groups: weekly irinotecan as single agent and irinotecan in combination with cisplatin/carboplatin plus concurrent radiation.

The studies from Kudoh et al. [30], Saka et al. [31] and Charkravarthy et al. [32] are comparably designed. Taken together, 60 patients received 30–60 mg/m^2 irinotecan weekly concurrently with a conventionally fractionated irradiation (2 Gy, total dose 60 Gy). There were 3 hematological side effects

KARGER

Fax +49 761 4 52 07 14
E-mail Information@Karger.de
www.karger.com

Accessible online at:
www.karger.com/journals/onk

G. Klautke
Universität Rostock
Klinik und Poliklinik für Strahlentherapie
Südring 75
D-18057 Rostock (Germany)

Tab. 1.

Author	Tumor type	Chemotherapy			Radiation	Response rate
		agent	schedule	mg/m²	Gy	
Koukourakis et al., 1999	head and neck cancer	docetaxel	weekly	20, 20, 25	2, 66, 70	
		cisplatin	day 1	25, 40, 55		CR: 9/12 – PR: 3/12
Kudoh et al., 1996	NSCLC, stage IIIa/b	irinotecan	weekly	30, 45, 60	2, 60	CR: 2 /24 – PR: 16/24
Saka et al., 1997	NSCLC, stage IIIa/b	irinotecan	weekly	60 2, 60		PR: 19/ 24
Chakravarthy et al., 1999	NSCLC, stage III	irinotecan	weekly	30, 40, 50	2, 40+20	PR: 7/ 12
Yokoyama et al., 1996	NSCLC, stage IIIa/b	irinotecan	day 1, 8, 15	40, 60		
		cisplatin	day 1, every 4 weeks, 3 courses	60, 60	2, 60	PR: 7/13
Nakagawa et al., 1997	NSCLC, stage IIIa/b	irinotecan	weekly	30, 40, 50		
		carboplatin	Mo–Fr	20	2, 60	CR: 2/23 – PR: 13/23
Klautke et al., 1999	NSCLC, stage IIIa/b	irinotecan	weekly	40		
		cisplatin	days 1–5 and 29–33	20	1,8, 50,4+12,6	CR: 2/10 – PR: 7/10
Mitchell et al., 1999	rectal cancer	irinotecan	days 1, 8, 15, 22	30–50		
		5-FU	Mo–Fr	300 /d, 225 /d	1,8, 45	CR: 5/20 R0-resection: 20/20
Minsky et al., 1999	rectal cancer	irinotecan	Mo–Fr in week 1, 2, 4, 5	8, 10, 13	1,8, 50,4	R0-resection: 17/17
Rostock	rectal cancer	irinotecan	weekly	40		
		5-FU	continuous	250 /d	1,8, 45+5,4	12 patients treated up to now, 6 patients operated, 5 R0-resection, CR:1/6

grade 3, and 6 patients had an esophagitis grade 3/4. Objective response rate was 73% (2/60 CR, 42/60 PR). The recommended dose of weekly irinotecan together with thoracic radiation was 40–45 mg/m². Remarkable in these trails was the relatively high rate of pneumonitis grade 3 (5/60), and 1 patient died of pneumonitis.

Yokoyama et al. [33] combined irinotecan (day 1, 8, 15) and cisplatin (60 mg/m², day 1). This schedule was repeated every 4 weeks for 3 courses. Concurrent radiotherapy (2 Gy/day up to 60 Gy) started with the 1st course of chemotherapy. The dose of irinotecan was escalated from 40 to 60 mg/m². The response rate of only 53% (7/13 PR) was caused by dose reduction or even termination of chemotherapy due to of leukopenia and fever. Moreover, radiotherapy was stopped in 3/13 patients before administering 40 Gy.

Nevertheless, Nakagawa et al. [34] and our own data [35] showed that it is possible to combine irinotecan and cisplatin or carboplatin effectively and safely with thoracic irradiation. Nakagawa applied irinotecan weekly (30, 40, 50 mg/m²) and carboplatin (20 mg/m²) from Monday to Friday over 6 weeks, concurrently with radiation (2 Gy/day up to 60 Gy). Response rate was 65% (2/23 CR, 13/23 PR). Only 1 pneumonitis grade 3 had to be recorded. In Rostock, 10 patients were treated with irinotecan (40 mg/m², weekly) and cisplatin (20 mg/m², days 1–5 and 29–33) simultaneously with thoracic irradiation (1.8 Gy/day up to 50.4 + 12.6 Gy). There were 2 leukopenia grade 3 and 1 thrombopenia grade 3, but no pneumonitis. Response rate was 90% (2/10 CR, histological confirmed; 7/10 PR).

Irinotecan has demonstrated particularly activity in patients with metastatic colorectal cancer. Nevertheless, the concurrent use of irinotecan and radiotherapy of the small pelvis was hesitated. Both modalities may cause diarrhea. The combined toxicity was thought to be very strong, possibly not to keep under control and life-threatening. This apprehension can be qualified by our own data and those of Mitchell et al. [36] and Minsky et al. [37].

Both groups treated preoperatively 24 and 17 patients, respectively, with locally advanced rectal cancer. Minsky et al. used a schedule of daily irinotecan (Monday to Friday: 8, 10, 13 mg/m²) in week 1, 2, 4, and 5 concurrently with irradiation of the small pelvis (1.8 Gy/day up to 50.4 Gy). The dose-limiting toxicities at a level of 13 mg/m² irinotecan were diarrhea and leukopenia. According to this trial, the recommended daily dose is 10 mg/m² irinotecan. All 17 patients had a complete resection of their tumors. Mitchell et al. [36] applied weekly irinotecan (30–50 mg/m²) and 5-fluorouracil (5-FU, 300 mg/m²; 225 mg/m² as continuous infusion) from Monday to Friday during radiotherapy (1.8 Gy/day up to 45 Gy). There was 1 leukopenia grade 4. Diarrhea was the dose-limiting toxicity. Up to now 20 patients were operated, 5/20 patients had a histological confirmed CR.

In Rostock, also 12 patients with locally advanced or recurrent rectal cancer were treated. Our schedule consisted of a weekly application of irinotecan (40 mg/m²); continuous infusion of 5-FU (250 mg/m²/day during radiation) simultaneously with radiotherapy (1.8 Gy/day up to 45 Gy + 5.4 Gy boost). There were 2/12 leukopenia grade 3 and 3/12 diarrhea grade 3 and 1/12 diarrhea grade 4. Up to now, 6 patients underwent surgery, 5 patients had a curative R0 resection; one tumor showed a histological confirmed CR. One patient, who refused surgery, attained a CR of her local recurrence, as shown by computed tomography. Another very interesting and important fact of this schedule is the high systemic activity on distant metastasis. One patient with pulmonary metastasis and 1 with liver metastasis showed a PR of this metastasis, although these regions were not irradiated.

Conclusions

The administration of irinotecan concurrently with irradiation shows promising results in patients with head and neck cancer, NSCLC, and rectal cancer. Moreover, these results warrant further clinical evaluation to define the level of toxicity and the activity of irinotecan and concurrent radiotherapy in other tumor types, like gastric, pancreatic or cervical cancer. Due to the small number of patients treated and the few investigations published, these schedules must be considered as an experimental therapy up to now. Therefore only skilled radio-oncologists should conduct further phase I/II trials to gain more patients and to define the role of radiotherapy-irinotecan in the treatment of individuals with these cancers. Nevertheless, the few possible serious side effects, such as febrile neutropenia, pneumonitis, violent diarrhea or enteritis, must be considered.

References

1 Hsiang YH, et al.: Arrest of replication forks by drug-stabilized topoisomerase-I-DNA cleavable complexes as a mechanism of cell killing by camptothecin. Cancer Res 1989;49:5077–5082.

2 Slichemyer WJ, et al.: The current status of camptothecin analogues as antitumor agents. J Natl Cancer Inst 1993;85:271–291.

3 Burris HA, Fields SM: Topoisomerase I inhibitors: An overview of the camptothecin analogs. Hematol Oncol Clin North Am 1994;8:333–355.

4 Pommier Y: Les ADN topo-isomérases, garde-barrières du génome et leur sabotage par les antibiotiques et les anticancéreux. Médicine Sciences 1994; 10:953–955.

5 Pommier Y, et al.: Cellular determinants of sensitivity and resistance to camptothecins; in Potmesil M, Pinedo H (eds): Camptothecins: New Anticancer Agents. Boka Raton, CRC Press, 1995.

6 Boothman DA, Trask DK, Pardee AB: Inhibition of potential lethal damage repair in human tumor cells by lapachone, an activator of topoisomerase I. Cancer Res. 1987;49:605–612.

7 Boscia RE, Korbut T, Holden SA, Teicher BA: Interaction of topoisomerase I inhibitors with radiation in cis-diamminedichloroplatinum(II)-sensitive and -resistant cells in vitro and in the FSAIIC fibrosarcoma in vivo. Int J Cancer 1993;53:118–123.

8 Omura M, Torigoe S, Kubota N: SN-38, a metabolite of the camptothecin derivative CPT-11, potentiates the cytotoxic effect of radiation in human colon adenocarcinoma cells grown as spheroids. Radiother Oncol 1997;43:197–201.

9 Rich TA, Kirichenko AV: Camptothecin radiation sensitization: Mechanisms, schedules, and timing. Oncology (New York) 1998;12:114–120.

10 Chen AY, Choy H, Rothenberg ML: DNA topoisomerase I-targeting drugs as radiation sensitizers. Oncology (Huntington) 1999;13:39–46.

11 Boige V, Raymond E, Fabbro M, et al.: Phase II trial and pharmacokinetic study of irinotecan (CPT-11) in patients with glioblastoma. Ann Oncol 1998;9(4):657.

12 Ilson DH, Saltz L, Enzinger P: Phase II trial of weekly irinotecan plus cisplatin in advanced esophageal cancer. J Clin Oncol 1999;17:3270–3275.

13 Shirao K, Shimada Y, Kondo H, et al.: Phase I–II study of irinotecan hydrochloride combined with cisplatin in patients with advanced gastric cancer. J Clin Oncol 1997;15:921–927.

14 Wagener DJ, Verdonk HE, Dirix LY, et al.: Phase II trial of CPT-11 in patients with advanced pancreatic cancer: An EORTC Early Clinical Trials Group study. Ann Oncol 1995;6:129–132.

15 Verschraegen CF, Levy T, Kudelka AP, et al.: Phase II study of irinotecan in prior chemotherapy-treated squamous cell carcinoma of the cervix. J Clin Oncol 1997;15:625–631.

16 Eisenhauer EA, Vermorken JB: New drugs in gynecologic oncology. Curr Opin Oncol 1996;8:408–414.

17 Mogi H, Hasegawa Y, Watanabe A, et al.: Combination effects of cisplatin, vinorelbine and irinotecan in non-small-cell lung cancer cell lines in vitro. Cancer Chemother Pharmacol 1997;39:199–204.

18 Adjei AA, Argiris A, Murren JR: Docetaxel and irinotecan, alone and in combination, in the treatment of non-small cell lung cancer. Sem Oncol 1999;26(suppl 16):32–40.

19 Kudoh S, Kurihara N, Okishio K, et al.: A phase I-II study of weekly irinotecan (CPT-11) and simultaneous thoracic radiotherapy for unresectable locally advanced non-small cell lung cancer. Proc Am Soc Clin Oncol 1996.

20 Lhomme C, Fumoleau P, Fargeot P, et al.: Results of a European Organization for Research and Treatment of Cancer / Early Clinical Studies Group phase II trial of first-line irinotecan in patients with advanced or recurrent squamous cell carcinoma of the cervix. J Clin Oncol 1999;17:3136–3142.

21 Irvin WP, Price FV, Bailey H, et al.: A phase II study of irinotecan (CPT-11) in patients with advanced squamous cell carcinoma of the cervix. Cancer 1998;82:328–333.

22 Look KY, Blessing JA, Levenback C, et al.: A phase II trial of VPT-11 in recurrent squamous carcinoma of the cervix: A gynecologic oncology group study. Gynecol Oncol 1998;70:334–338.

23 DeVore RF, Johnson DH, Crawford J, et al.: Phase II study of irinotecan plus cisplatin in patients with advanced non-small-cell lung cancer. J Clin Oncol 1999;17:2710–2720.

24 van Cutsem E, Cunningham D, ten Bokkel Huinink W, et al.: Irinotecan (CPT-11) multicenter phase II study in colorectal cancer patients with documented progressive disease on prior 5-FU: preliminary results. Proc Ann Meet Soc Clin Oncol 1996;15:562(abstr).

25 Droz JP, Marty M, Douillard JP, et al.: CPT-11 in 5-FU-resistant colorectal cancer: Management of delayed diarrhoea. Ann Oncol 1996;7(suppl 3):223P.

28 Shimada Y, et al.: Phase II study of CPT-11, a new camptothecin derivative, in metastatic colorectal cancer (ENG). J Clin Oncol 1993;11:909–913.

27 Pilot HC, Wender MJ, O'Connel, et al.: A phase II trial of CPT-11 (irinotecan) in patients with metastatic colorectal carcinoma: A North Central Cancer Treatment Group (NCCTG) study. Proc Ann Meet Am Soc Clin Oncol 1994;13:abstr 573.

28 Cunningham D, Pyrhönen S, James RD, et al.: A phase III multicenter randomized study of CPT-11 versus supportive care alone in patients with 5-FU-resistant metastatic colorectal colorectal cancer. Proc Ann Meet Am Soc Clin Oncol 1998;17:abstr 1.

29 Koukourakis MI, Bizakis JG, Skoulakis CE, et al.: Combined irinotecan, docetaxel and conventionally fractionated radiotherapy in locally advanced head and neck cancer. A phase I dose escalation study. Anticancer Res 1999;19:2305–2309.

30 Kudoh S, Fujiwara Y, Takada Y, et al.: Phase II study of irinotecan combined with cisplatin in patients with previously untreated small-cell lung cancer. J Clin Oncol 1998;16:1068–1074.

31 Saka H, Shimokata K, Yoshida S, et al.: Irinotecan (CPT-11) and concurrent radiotherapy in locally advanced non-small cell lung cancer (NSCLC): A phase II study of Japan Clinical Oncology Group (JCOG9504). Proc Ann Meet Am Soc Clin Oncol 1997;16A:1607.

32 Chakravarthy A, Choy H, DeVore RF, et al.: Phase I trial of outpatient weekly irinotecan and concurrent radiation therapy for stage II unresectable non-small-cell lung cancer: A Vanderbilt Cancer Center Affiliate Network (VCCAN) Trial. 35th ASCO Ann Meet 1999; May 15–18, p 259, abstr. 1924.

33 Yokoyama A, Kurita K, Saijo N, et al.: Phase I/II study of irinotecan (CPT-1) and cisplatin plus concurrent thoracic radiation therapy in stage III non-small cell lung cancer: A Japan Clinical Oncology Group (JCOG) trial. Proc Am Soc Clin Oncol 1996;15:407(abstr 1242).

34 Nakagawa, K, Yamamoto N, Kudoh S, et al.: Irinotecan (CPT-11) and carboplatin (CBDCA) with concurrent thoracic radiotherapy (TRT) for unresectable, stage III non-small cell lung cancer (NSCLC) -preliminary results. 34th Ann. Meeting Am Soc Clin Oncol 1998, May 15–20, abstr 1909.

35 Klautke G, Peters K, Papuga C, Fietkau R: Simultane Radiochemotherapie mit Irinotecan und Cisplatin beim NSCLC. Strahlenther Onkol 1999;175 (suppl 1):41.

36 Mitchell E, Ahmad N, Fry R, et al.: Combined modality therapy of locally advanced or recurrent adenocarcinoma of the rectum: Preliminary report of a phase I trial of chemotherapy (CT) with CPT-11, 5-FU and concomitant irradiation (RT). 35th ASCO Ann Meet 1999, May 15–18, abstr 948.

37 Minsky BD, O'Reilly E, Wong D, et al.: Daily low-dose irinotecan (CPT-11) plus pelvic irradiation as preoperative treatment of locally advanced rectal cancer. 35th ASCO Ann Meet 1999, May 15–18, abstr 1023.

ONKOLOGIE

Onkologie 2000;23(suppl 4):34–36

Options for Treatment of Lung Cancer with Irinotecan

U. Gatzemeier

Zentrum für Pneumologie und Thoraxchirurgie, Krankenhaus Großhansdorf

Introduction

In Germany, around 45,000 individuals are diagnosed with lung cancer each year. Considering the current 5-year survival rate of approximately 13%, the prognosis is still extremely unsatisfactory. A new strategy for improving the treatment results, even in advanced, inoperable tumor stages, comprises the introduction of new drugs. Irinotecan, a topoisomerase I inhibitor, is a such new substance which was investigated in recent years in both small-cell and non-small cell lung cancer.

Non-Small Cell Lung Cancer

Therapeutic nihilism is no longer justified in non-small cell lung cancer (NSCLC). In recent years, a number of meta-analyses and randomized clinical studies have shown that various chemotherapy regimens, especially those including platinum, are now capable of extending survival, even in patients with inoperable non-small cell lung cancer. Furthermore, they are superior in controlling symptoms and can increase the quality of life compared to the 'best supportive care' alone. When left untreated, the median survival in patients with metastatic NSCLC is 4–6 months, and the 1-year survival rate is about 10%. The use of chemotherapy combinations containing cisplatin makes it possible to achieve remission rates of 20–30%, a median survival of 6–8 months, and 1-year survival of about 20–25%.
New substances, such as taxanes, gemcitabines and vinorelbines, produced remission rates of over 20% when used alone. The 1-year survival achieved when these new substances were used in combination chemotherapy was reported to be 30–40% in various phase II and III studies.

Phase II Studies with Irinotecan

The findings of three studies of irinotecan in previously untreated patients with advanced non-small cell lung cancer have now been published (table 1). These studies demonstrated that irinotecan has significant activity in advanced non-small cell lung cancer. Consequently, combination chemotherapies with irinotecan were also investigated in phase II trials.
Irinotecan was utilized in combination with cisplatin in the majority of studies published up to now (table 2). The authors administered different dosages, using 60–70 mg/m^2 of irinotecan on days 1, 8 and 15 and 160 mg/m^2 on day 1, repeated every 4 weeks. Cisplatin was normally given in doses of 80 mg/m^2 on day 1, repeated every 4 weeks. In some studies, the cisplatin dose was also split into 2-, 3- or 5-day partial doses (table 2). The remission rates in patients treated with a combination of irinotecan and cisplatin ranged from 28–58%. A median survival of 9.9 months was achieved by De Vore [6], and Ueoka [9] even achieved a rate of 13 months. In the studies where indicated, the 1-year survival ranged from 33 to 58%. These rates are certainly equal to those achieved using the so-called novel modern chemotherapy combinations. The dose-limiting symptoms observed in all these studies were WHO grade 3–4 leukopenia in up to 49% of cases and WHO grade 3–4 diarrhea in up to 27%.
Other combinations under investigation at present combine irinotecan with taxanes (docetaxel or paclitaxel), gemcitabine, mitomycine C, or vinorelbine.

Phase III Studies

The first two phase III studies incorporating irinotecan in the treatment of advanced non-small cell lung cancer were published at ASCO 1999 (table 3). Niho [11] tested a combination consisting of 60 mg/m^2 irinotecan on days 1, 8, 15 and 80 mg/m^2 cisplatin on day 1 in cycles repeated every 4 weeks compared to a combination of cisplatin and vindesine. The findings in a total of 190 treated patients revealed a slightly better remission rate for the irinotecan-cisplatin combination. There was no significant difference between irinotecan-cisplatin (45 weeks) and vindesine-cisplatin (49 weeks) with respect to the median survival.

KARGER

Fax +49 761 4 52 07 14
E-mail Information@Karger.de
www.karger.com

Accessible online at:
www.karger.com/journals/onk

Dr. U. Gatzemeier
Krankenhaus Großhansdorf
Zentrum für Pneumologie und Thoraxchirurgie
Wöhrendamm 80
D-22927 Großhansdorf (Germany)

Table 1. Treatment of NSCLC with irinotecan alone

Author	Dose, mg/m^2	Scheme	Patients, N	Remission, %	Median survival, months
Negoro [1]	100	weekly 3/4	67	34	not specified
Fukuoka [2]	100	weekly	72	32	10.5
Baker [3]	100	weekly 4/6	48	16	6.2

Table 2. Treatment of advanced NSCLC with a combination of irinotecan and cisplatin

Author	Irinotecan		Cisplatin		Patients, N	Remission, %	Median survival, months	1-year survival, %
	dose, mg/m^2	scheme	dose, mg/m^2	scheme				
Masuda [4]	60	days 1, 8, 15	80	day 1	69	52	–	33
Nakagawa [5]	60	days 1, 8, 15	80	day 1	69	48	–	–
De Vore [6]	60	days 1, 8, 15	80	day 1	52	28.9	9.9	not specified
Wagner [7]	70	days 1, 8, 15	40	days 1, 8, 15	35	31	–	not specified
Mori [8]	160	day 1	20	days 1–5	41	8.5	10.4	44
Ueoko [9]	50	days 1, 8	60	days 1, 8	42	51	13.0	58

Table 3. Phase III study of irinotecan in advanced NSCLC

Author	Agent	Dose, mg/m^2	Scheme	Patients, N	Remission, %	Median survival, weeks	1-year survival, %
Niho [11]	irinotecan	60	days 1, 8, 15	98	29	45.4	–
	cisplatin	80	day 1				
			4-week cycles				
	vinorelbine	3	days 1, 8, 15	101	22	49.6	–
	cisplatin	80	day 1				
			4-week cycles				
Masuda [12]	irinotecan	60	days 1, 8, 15	128	43	50.3	47.5
	cisplatin	80	day 1				
			4-week cycles				
	vinorelbine	3	days 1, 8, 15	123	31	47.4	37.9
	cisplatin	80	day 1				
			4-week cycles				
	irinotecan	100	days 1, 8, 15	124	21	46.1	40.7

Table 4. Treatment of SCLC with irinotecan alone

Author	Dose, mg/m^2	Scheme	Patients	Remission, %	Prior treatment
Negoro [13]	100	weekly	27	33.3	+
Masuda [14]	100	weekly 4/6	15	47	+
Le Chevalier [15]	350	3-week cycles	32	16	+
De Vore [16]	125	weekly 4/6	44	16	+

Table 5. Treatment of SCLC using combination chemotherapy with irinotecan

Author	Irinotecan		Combo CT		Patients, N	Remission, %	Prior therapy
	dose, mg/m^2	scheme	agent, mg/m^2	scheme			
Fujiwara [18]	60–80	days 1, 8, 15	cisplatin, 60	day 1	32	79	–
Okishio [17]	60	days 1, 8, 15	cisplatin, 60	day 1	16	19	+
Masuda [19]	70	days 1, 8, 15	etoposide, 80	days 1–3	25	71	+

The second study, published by Masuda, utilized a 3-arm prospective study design to compare an irinotecan/cisplatin combination with a vindesine/cisplatin combination and with irinotecan alone, using doses of 100 mg/m^2 on days 1, 8 and 15. A total of 375 patients were treated. The remission rate for the irinotecan/cisplatin combination was 43% compared to 31% for the vindesine/cisplatin combination and 21% for irinotecan alone. The irinotecan/cisplatin combination also achieved a significantly better 1-year survival rate (47.5%) than the vindesine/cisplatin combination (37.9%) and irinotecan alone (40.7%).

Small-Cell Lung Cancer

Small-cell bronchogenic carcinomas are chemosensitive tumors. A number of active substances can be used to treat them. The activity of the so-called novel drugs is also comparable to that of the already established substances.

The published findings regarding the use of irinotecan alone for treatment of pretreated small-cell lung cancer were obtained in four studies so far (table 4). On the whole, these four studies clearly demonstrate the activity of irinotecan alone in patients with previously treated small-cell lung cancer.

Additional studies in which irinotecan was combined with drugs such as cisplatin and etoposide are described in table 5.

Summary

Irinotecan is a substance with reliable activity in both small-cell and non-small cell lung cancers. Remission rates of 29–58% can be achieved in patients with non-small cell bronchogenic carcinomas treated with a combination of irinotecan and cisplatin. This is comparable to the data published for the other so-called novel substances combined with cisplatin. These rates were consistently achieved in various phase II studies using irinotecan doses of 60–80 mg/m^2 and cisplatin doses of 60–80 mg/m^2.

Phase I/II studies of irinotecan combined with other novel active substances have been initiated. The first phase III studies show a slight superiority of irinotecan and cisplatin compared to the former standard cisplatin/vindesine combinations. Nonetheless, further phase III studies will be needed to define the value of irinotecan in non-small cell lung cancer.

Irinotecan also has significant activity in small-cell lung cancer. Phase III studies will also be required to determine the definitive value of irinotecan in this cancer entity.

References

1 Negoro S, Fukuoka M, Niitani H, et al: A phase II study of CPT-11, a camptothecin derivative, in patients with primary lung cancer. Jpn J Cancer Chemother 1991;18:1013–1019.

2 Fukuoka M, Niitani H, Suzuki A, et al: A Phase II study of CPT-11, a new derivative of captothecin, for previously untreated non-small cell lung cancer. J Clin Oncol 1992;10:16–20.

3 Baker L, Khan R, Lynch T, Savaraj N, Sandler A, Feun L, Schaser R, Hanover C, Petit R: Phase II study of irinotecan in advanced non-small cell lung cancer (NSCLC). Proc Am Soc Clin Oncol 1997;16: 461a(abstr 1658).

4 Masuda N; Fukuoka M, Jujita A, Kurita Y, Tsuchiya S, Nagao K, Negoro S, Nishikaqa H, Katakami N, Nakagawa K, Niitani H: A phase II trial of combination of CPT-11 and Cisplatin for advanced non-small cell lung cancer. Br J Cancer 1998;78:251–256.

5 Nakagawa K, Fukuoka M, Niitani H: Phase II study of irinotecan (CPT-11) and cisplatin in patients with advanced non-small cell lung cancer. Proc Am Soc Clin Oncol 1993;12:1104(abstr).

6 Devore R, Johnson D, Crawford J, Dimery I, Eckhardt J, Eckhardt SG: Irinotecan plus cisplatin in patients with advanced non-small cell lung cancer. An overview of phase II trial results. Oncology 1998;12(suppl 6):79–83.

7 Wagner H, Faderl B, Dankelmann E, Deuss B, Achterrath W, v. Pawel J: Phase II study of irinotecan in combination with cisplatin as first line chemotherapy in advanced non small cell lung cancer (NSCLC). Proc Am Soc Clin Oncol 1999;18: 2032(abstr).

8 Mori K, Machida S, Yoshida T, Yoshida M, Kano Y, Tominaga K: A phase II study of irinotecan and infusional cisplatin with recombinant human granulocyte colony-stimulating factor support for advanced non-small cell lung cancer. Cancer Chemother Pharmacol 1999;43:467–470.

9 Ueoka H, Kiura K, Hiraki S, Eguchi K, Okimoto N, Harita S, Marukawa M, Yonei T, Kamei H, Segawa Y, Shibayama T, Harada M: Fractionated administration of Cisplatin (CDDP) and Irinotecan (CPT-11) in patients with stage IIIB and IV non-small cell lung Cancer (NSCLC): A phase II study. Proc Am Soc Clin Oncol 1999;18:2026(abstr).

10 Oshita F, Noda K, Nishiwaki Y, Fujita A, K, Kurita Y, Nakabayashi T, Tobise K, Abe S, Suzuki S, Hayashi I, Kawakami Y, Matsuda T, Tsuchiya S, Takahashi S, Tamura T, Saijo N: Phase-II study of irinotecan and etoposide in patients with metastatic non-small cell lung cancer. J Clin Oncol 1999; 15:304–309.

11 Niho S, Nagao K, Nishiwaki Y, Yokoyama A, Saijo N, Ohashi Y Niitani H and the CPT-11 Lung Cancer Study Group: Randomized multicenter phase III trial of irinotecan (CPT-11) and cisplatin (CDDP) versus CDDP and vindesine (VDS) in patients with advanced non-small cell lung cancer (NSCLC). Proc Am Soc Clin Oncol 1999;18: 1897(abstr).

12 Masuda N, Fukuoka M, Negoro S, Takada Y, Sugiura T, Ohashi Y, Ariyoshi Y, Niitani H and the CPT-11 Lung Cancer Study Group West: Randomized trial comparing Cisplatin (CDDP) and Irinotecan (CPT-11) vs. CCCP and vindesine (VDS) vs. CPT-11 alone in advanced NSCL, a multicenter phase III study. Proc Am Soc Clin Oncol 1999;18:1774(abstr).

13 Negoro S, Fukuoka M, Niitani H, et al: A phase II study of CPT-11, a camptothecin derivative, in patients with primary lung cancer. Jpn J Cancer Chemother 1991;18:1013–1019.

14 Masuda N, Fukuoka M, Kusunoki Y et al: CPT-11: A new derivative of camptothecin for the treatment of refractory or relapsed small-cell lung cancer. J Clin Oncol 1992;10:1225–1229.

15 Le Chevalier T, Ibrahim N, Chomy P, Riviere A, Monnier A, Magherini E, Pujol JL: A phase II study of irinotecan (CPT-11) in patients (pts) with small cell lung cancer (SCLC) progressing after initial response to first-line chemotherapy (CT). Proc Am Soc Clin Oncol 1997;16:A1617.

16 De Vore R, Blanke C, Denham C, Hainsworth J, Gralla R, Koletsky,Savaraj N, Vogel C, Sarna G, Brook D, Petit R, Elfring G, Schaaf L, Hanover C, Miller L: Phase II study of irinotecan (CPT-11) in patients with previously treated small-cell lung cancer (SCLC). Proc Am Soc Clin Oncol 1999;18: 1736(abstr).

17 Okishio K, Furuse K, Kawahara M, Ogawara M, Atagi S, Kawaguchi T, Tsuchiyama T: A phase II study of irinotecan (CPT-11) and cisplatin (CDDP) in previously treated small cell lung cancer (SCLC). Proc Am Soc Clin Oncol 1998;17:1914(abstr).

18 Masuda N, Matsui K, Negoro S, et al: Combination of irinotecan and etoposide for treatment of refractory or relapsed small-cell lung cancer. J Clin Oncol 1998;16;3329–3334.

19 Masuda N, Matsui K, Negoro S, Takifuji N, Takeda K, Yana T, Kobayashi M, Hirashima T, Kusunoki Y, Ushijima S, Kawase I, Tada T, Sawaguchi H, Fukuoka M: Combination of irinotecan and etoposide for treatment of refractory or relapsed small-cell lung cancer. J Clin Oncol 1998;16:3329–3334.

ONKOLOGIE

Onkologie 2000;23(suppl 4):37–38

Treatment of Gynecological Carcinomas with Campto®

J.-U. Blohmer W. Lichtenegger

Klinik für Frauenheilkunde und Geburtshilfe, Campus Charité-Mitte, Medizinische Fakultät der Humboldt-Universität zu Berlin

Invasive cervical carcinoma is the 5th most common form of cancer worldwide and takes 2nd place as the leading tumor-related cause of death in women [1]. In Germany, approximately 7000 new cases are treated each year [2]. Apart from a 40% reduction in the overall incidence of carcinoma of the cervix, an increasing prevalence of cervical cancer has been observed in younger women over the past 20 years or so [3].

The results of treatment of FIGO stage IA-IIA tumors are generally excellent. In the presence of more unfavorable prognostic factors, such as lymph node metastasis, lymph vessel invasion, and parametrial tumor invasion, the results of treatment are still just as unsatisfactory as they have been for decades (5-year survival rate of 53–70%).

The treatment results are especially poor in women with more advanced tumors (IIIB-IVB) and a recurrence of cervical cancer. In these patients, the 5-year survival rate is <5–28% [4]. The introduction of new treatment options for advanced cervical cancer is therefore urgently needed. This can include new chemotherapeutic agents such as irinotecan (Campto®).

The standard agent for first- and second-line chemotherapy of advanced cervical carcinoma is currently cisplatin (50–100 mg/m^2), which achieves a response rate of 17–31% [5].

Irinotecan was able to achieve a median response rate of 18% (95% CI: 11–26%) in conjunction with a median progression-free survival of 4 months and a median overall survival of 6 months in platinum-pretreated females with cervical cancer (four phase II studies in a total of 120 patients) [6].

The combination of irinotecan with the established agent cisplatin is very promising. A median response rate of 78% (95% CI: 58–90%) was achieved in a phase II study in 23 patients with locally advanced and recurrent cervical cancer. The following dosage was used: irinotecan (60 mg/m^2) on days 1, 8 and 15 plus cisplatin (60 mg/m^2) on day 1; the treatment was repeated every 4 weeks, with a dose density of 45 mg/m^2 irinotecan and 15 mg/m^2 cisplatin per week [7].

These excellent findings are supported by a phase II study of neoadjuvant treatment of locally advanced cervical cancer (25 female patients, stages IB2–IIIB, squamous cell carcinomas) in which a median response rate of 80% (95% CI: 61–91%) and a 12% rate of complete remission was achieved. The therapy regimen was as follows: irinotecan (60 mg/m^2) on days 1, 8, 15 plus cisplatin (60 mg/m^2) on day 1, repeated every 4 weeks for a total of 2 or 3 cycles. Of the 56 treatment cycles administered, grade 3 or 4 neutropenia was observed in 75% and grade 3–4 diarrhea in 10%; there were no therapy-related deaths [8].

Verweij et al. [9] examined a less expensive irinotecan-cisplatin regimen for chemotherapy of cervical cancer in a phase I study using irinotecan (300 mg/m^2) plus cisplatin (60 mg/m^2), repeated every 3 weeks. Febrile neutropenia and diarrhea were the dose-limiting effects. Doses of 200 mg/m^2 irinotecan plus 50 mg/m^2 cisplatin could be administered every 3 weeks without causing severe toxicity. The weekly dose density was 67 mg/m^2 irinotecan and 17 mg/m^2 cisplatin, respectively.

Based on this study, H. Kuehnle and W. Lichtenegger now plan to carry out a phase III study in Germany to compare the results of treatment of metastatic and recurrent cervical cancer with 50 mg/m^2 of cisplatin on day 1, repeated every 3 weeks, versus 200 mg/m^2 of irinotecan on day 1, repeated every 3 weeks, in combination with cisplatin 50 mg/m^2. The primary goal of the study is to compare the progression-free survival time achieved with cisplatin monotherapy to that achieved with irinotecan-cisplatin combination chemotherapy.

The activity of irinotecan in ovarian cancer is comparable to that of other topoisomerase I inhibitors. In phase I and II studies, response rates of 16–30% were achieved using irinotecan alone; rates of 40–60% where achieved when the drug was combined with platinum or mitomycin (especially in cases of platinum- and taxane-resistant clear cell carcinomas of the ovary) [10, 11].

KARGER

Fax +49 761 4 52 07 14
E-mail Information@Karger.de
www.karger.com

Accessible online at:
www.karger.com/journals/onk

Dr. med. Jens-Uwe Blohmer
Klinik für Frauenheilkunde und Geburtshilfe, Campus Charité-Mitte
Medizinische Fakultät der Humboldt-Universität zu Berlin
Schumannstraße 20/21
D-10117 Berlin (Germany)

References

1 Parkin DM, Laara E, Muir CS: Estimates of the worldwide frequency of sixteen major cancer 1980. Int J Cancer 1988;41:184–197.

2 Becker N, Wahrendorf J: Krebsatlas der Bundesrepublik Deutschland 1981–1990. Berlin, Springer 1998.

3 Luschin-Ebengreuth G: Cervical cancer. Prognostic factors. Age; in Burghardt E, Webb MJ, Monaghan JM, Kindermann G (eds): Surgical Gynecologic Oncology. Stuttgart, Thieme, 1993, pp 322–324.

4 Omura GA; Blessing JA; Vaccarello L; Berman ML; Clarke-Pearson DL; Mutch DG; Anderson: Randomized trial of cisplatin versus cisplatin plus mitolactol versus cisplatin plus ifosfamide in advanced squamous carcinoma of the cervix: A Gynecologic Oncology Group study. J Clin Oncol 1997; 15:165–171.

5 Bonomi P, Blessing JA, Stehman FB, DiSaia PJ, Walton L, Major FJ: Randomized trial of three cisplatin dose schedules in squamous-cell carcinoma of the cervix: A Gynecologic Oncology Group study. J Clin Oncol 1985;3:1079–1085.

6 Verschraegen CF, Levy T, Kudelka AP, Llerena E, Ende K, Freedman RS, Edwards CL, Hord M, Steger M, Kaplan AL, Kieback D, Fishman A, Kavanagh JJ: Phase II study of irinotecan in prior chemotherapy-treated squamous cell carcinoma of the cervix. J Clin Oncol 1997;15:625–631.

7 Sugiyama T, Nishida T, Kumagai S, Nishio S, Fujiyoshi K, Okura N, Yakushiji M, Hiura M, Umesaki N: Combination therapy with irinotecan and cisplatin as neoadjuvant chemotherapy in locally advanced cervical cancer. Br J Cancer 1999;81:95–98.

8 Kumagai S, Sugiyama T, Fujiyoshi K, Nishida T, Yakushiji M, Hiura M, Umesaki V: Combination therapy with irinotecan and cisplatin as neoadjuvant chemotherapy in locally advanced cervical cancer. Proc Am Soc Clin Oncol 1999;abstr 1458.

9 Verweij J, deJonge MJA, Sparreboom A, Planting AST, van der Burg MEL, de Boer-Dennert MM, ter Steeg J, Jaques C, Soter G: Phase I and pharmacokinetic (Pk) study of irinotecan (CPT-11) and cisplatin (C) in patients with solid tumors. Proc Am Soc Clin Oncol 1998;abstr 724.

10 Rosen LS: Irinotecan in lymphoma, leukemia, and breast, pancreatic, ovarian, and small-cell lung cancers. Oncology (Huntingt) 1998;12(suppl 6):103–109.

11 Verschraegen CF, Kudelka AP, Kavanagh JJ: Topoisomerase-I inhibitors in gynaecologic tumours. Ann Acad Med Singapore 1998;27:683–687.

ONKOLOGIE

Onkologie 2000;23

Guidelines for Authors

ONKOLOGIE is a peer-reviewed journal intended to provide a forum for presentation of all aspects of oncology, including reviews and original articles from internal hematology and oncology, surgical, gynecological and urological oncology, radiation therapy as well as clinical-experimental oncology. Contributions to pediatric, ENT and dermatological oncology, pathology, biometry, epidemiology, prevention, early diagnosis and psychological care will also be considered.

1. General Information and Publishing Rights

Manuscripts for publication should be submitted in quadruplicate (each copy accompanied by a complete set of figures and tables) to S. Karger Publishers, attn.: Dr. Heike Endemann, Postfach, D-79095 Freiburg. Each author should always keep a copy of the manuscript.

In a **covering** letter all authors must confirm with their signature that the submitted paper or parts of it (with the exception of congress reports) were not previously published and are not submitted for publication elsewhere. All authors have to confirm that they have read the manuscript and agree to have it published in the submitted form. It is the authors' responsibility to obtain permission from other publishers to reproduce illustrations, tables, etc. Acceptance of a manuscript is based on the evaluation by several reviewers (peer review). Once the manuscript is accepted for publication, all rights are retained by the publisher. The publication, or parts of it, may neither be translated into other languages nor reproduced by any mechanical or electronic means (including photocopying, recording, and microfilm) nor stored in a retrieval system without the publisher's written permission.

Ethical and Legal Prerequisites: Manuscripts involving examinations of probands and patients must include a statement that the trial protocol has been approved by an ethical committee and thus meets the standards of the Declaration of Helsinki in its revised version of 1975 and its amendments made in 1983, 1989, and 1996 [JAMA 1997;277:925–926]. Accordingly, the proband's informed consent has to be included in the manuscript. Information suitable to reveal the proband's identity is to be avoided. Experiments involving animals demand consent as well and must meet the requirements of current German laws for the protection of animals. A reference to this approval must be included in the manuscript. Articles from countries other than Germany must include a comparable note.

Categories: Contributions are classified as Review Article, Short Review, Original Article, Ongoing Clinical Trial, FAX Communication, Short Communication, Casuistic Contribution, Clinical-Pathological Conference, Letter to the Editors, Commentary, Opinion, Oncological Education, Clinical Information or Congress Report, or Wilsede School. Review articles, original articles, ongoing clinical trials, FAX communications, short communications, casuistic contributions, letters to the editors, commentaries and articles on clinical-pathological conferences must be written in English (American or British spelling and grammar). All other contributions may be submitted either in German or in English.

2. Preparation of Manuscripts

Please print the manuscript 1¹/₂-spaced with 3-cm margins (left and right). The text (including the summary) should be limited to 10 manuscript pages for review articles, 8 pages for short reviews and original articles, 6 pages for other contributions. Tables, figures, and references are not included Each additional complete or partial page to print may be charged to the author (see below). Please check the final copy carefully for consistent notations and correct spelling. Accepted manuscripts are edited according to the publisher's style. General information for the preparation of manuscripts may be found in 'Uniform Requirements for Manuscripts Submitted to Biomedical Journals' by the International Committee of Medical Journal Editors as published in Ann Intern Med 1997;126:36–47 (available from: www.asma-assn.org/public/journals/jama/sc6336.htm).

Electronic Manuscript Submission: Each manuscript must be accompanied by a disk exactly matching the printed version. Please see 'Guidelines for Electronic Manuscript Submission' in the first issue of each volume for assistance in preparing manuscripts on disk.

All pages should be numbered consecutively, starting with the title page. Articles should be structured as follows: **Key Words and Summary, Schlüsselwörter** and **Zusammenfassung, Introduction, Material and Methods (**optionally **Patients and Methods), Results, Discussion,** optionally **Acknowledgements, References, tables, figure legends,** and **figures.**

The **title page** must include the following information: Title and short title in English and German, each author's full name, followed by hospital, institute, etc.; exact postal address of the corresponding author including phone and fax numbers as well as E-mail address.

Original articles must contain an English **and** a German (translation by the editor is possible) **structured summary** (for more information refer to Haynes RB, Mulrow CD, Huth EJ, Altman DG, Gardner MJ: Ann Intern Med 1990;113:69–76) of not more than 250 words in four paragraphs: **Background, Material and Methods, Results, Conclusions.** Summaries should not include any references, tables, figures, or references to figures and tables. If it is inevitable to cite a reference, complete publication data must be given. Each article must have 3–5 **key words** (English and German). If possible, use terms from the Medical Subject Headings List (MeSH) of Index Medicus (available at www.nlm.nih.gov). Review articles do not adhere to the framework of original articles; however, the title page, summaries, key words, and a list of references are necessary.

Footnotes should be used only for tables. Please use **abbreviations** as economically as possible. Special abbreviations should be written in full when first mentioned, followed by the abbreviation in parentheses, e. g. adenosine monophosphate (AMP). When first mentioned, **registered trade names** must be marked with the superscript registration symbol ® or ™. It is the sole responsibility of the author to ensure that this rule is followed properly.

Acknowledgements should be placed directly after the text and before the list of references.

The list of **references** should include only the publications cited in the text. References must be numbered sequentially in the order cited in the text, do not alphabetize. Insert textual references in square brackets. In each reference all authors should be mentioned; the abbreviation 'et al.' is to be avoided. It is recommended to quote only articles already published or accepted for publication. Please avoid notices like 'in preparation' or 'personal communication'. Authors are responsible for the accuracy and completeness of their references and for correct text citation. The journal titles should be abbreviated according to the Index Medicus system (www.nlm.nih.gov). For references, please follow the examples given:

(a) Papers published in periodicals: Lelie PN, Cuypers HTM, van Drimmelen AAJ, Quint WGV: Quality assessment of hepatitis C virus nucleic acid amplification methods. An international proficiency study. Infusionsther Transfusionsmed 1998;25:102–110.

(b) Edited books: Hardy WD Jr, Essex M: FeLV-induced feline acquired immune deficiency syndrome: A model for human AIDS; in Klein E (ed): Acquired Immunodeficiency Syndrome. Prog Allergy. Basel, Karger, 1986, vol 37, pp 353–376.

(c) Monographs: Schaefer UW, Beelen DW: Bone Marrow Transplantation, ed 2, revised. Basel, Karger, 1996.

The number of **figures** and **tables** should be kept low. They are listed in the text as (fig. 1) and (table 1). Data explained in tables need not be repeated in the text. Figure legends must be listed together on a separate page. Figure and table legends should be kept short and precise. **Color illustrations** are reproduced at the author's expense (see below).

Figures should be submitted in quadruplicate, 1 original and 3 copies. Please do not fasten them, and mark on the back the first author's name, a short form of the title, the 'top' instruction, and the number of the figure. The quality of the illustrations printed depends on the quality of the originals provided.

Reports on Randomized Controlled Trials (RCTs) should be prepared according to the CONSORT statement [Begg C, Cho M, Eastwood S, Horton S, Moher D, Olki I, Pitkin R, Rennie D, Schulz F, Simel D, Stroup D: Improving the quality of reporting of randomized trials: The CONSORT statement. JAMA 1996;276:637–639].The report must state explicitly how the comparison groups were assembled, allowing the reader to access the method of randomization. Please specify in the title and summary that the manuscript is a report on an RCT. When an RCT is submitted, the authors should refer to the checklist 'Checklist for Authors Submitting Randomized Controlled Trials' reprinted in the guidelines of the first issue of a volume. Checklist and flow diagram are also available at: www.ama-assn.org/public/journals/jama. Both should be submitted with the manuscript, as they will be included in the review process.

Galley Proofs: The edited manuscript and the galley proofs are forwarded together with a reprint order form to the corresponding author. The author is asked to verify the galleys against the manuscript and to mark appropriate corrections in the galley proofs. Correspondence regarding accepted manuscripts and proofs should be directed to the publisher.

3. Costs and Reprints

a) The author will be charged for corrections to the galley proofs entailing expenses in excess of 10% of the original typesetting costs.
b) If a paper exceeds the allotted size and will not be abridged by the author, each additional printed page is charged to the author at DEM 650.00.
c) Color illustrations are reproduced at the author's expense. Each is charged to the author at DEM 450.00 as a contribution to the additional reproduction and color printing costs.

The corresponding author will receive 25 reprints free of charge.

The complete guidelines are printed in the first issue of each volume.

KARGER

Fax +49 761 4 52 07 14
E-mail Information@Karger.de
www.karger.com

Guidelines for Authors available at:
www.karger.com/journals/onk/onk_gl.htm

ONKOLOGIE

Onkologie 2000;23

Guidelines for Electronic Manuscript Submission

The final version of the manuscript must be accompanied by a disk **exactly** matching the printed version. Check the disk with a virus detection program. Do not use programs for file compression. Label the disk with the title of the manuscript, the first author, the platform, and the version of software used. We accept disks in Macintosh or MS-DOS (Windows) format. When preparing a manuscript, use the document mode or its equivalent in the word-processing program. If a non-Western version of the word-processing program is used to prepare the manuscript, save the text in the rich-text format (RTF). The preferred word-processing package is MS-Word. Other commonly used text programs and ASCII formats are accepted.

In the file do not include any layout instructions such as placements for graphics. The text should be justified to the left, and end-of-line hyphenation should be avoided. Use carriage returns only to end heading and paragraphs, not to break lines of text. Use only **one format** (normal) for the document; to structure the text you may use tabs. Please do not include any headers, footers, or footnotes. Ensure that all characters are correctly represented throughout the manuscript: e.g., 1 (one) and l (ell), 0 (zero) and O (Oh), X (ex) and × (times sign). Please save tables and figures each as separate files, do **not** integrate them in the text (see also 'Figures'). The use of the fonts Times and Symbol is recommended.

Figures

Graphics, e.g. figures, schemes, etc., should be saved as separate files. Most packages for creating them will allow the user to choose a format in which to save a file. TIFF, PostScript, or EPS is preferred. It should be possible to identify the figure by the filename. All figures **must** be submitted additionally as camera-ready copies.

References

Use the style as described in 'Guidelines for Authors', i.e., no comma after the last name, no period after the initials. The semicolon and colon after the year of publication and the volume number, respectively, should not be followed by spaces before volume number and page number. Please give the first and the last page of the article, separated by a dash. *Wrong:* Infusionsther Transfusionsmed 1998; 25: 160 – 3., *correct:* Infusionsther Transfusionsmed 1998;25:160–163.

Hinweise für Manuskripte auf Diskette

Bitte reichen Sie zusammen mit dem angenommenen Manuskript eine Diskette ein. Prüfen Sie die Diskette mit einem Virensuchprogramm. Der Inhalt der Diskette **muß exakt** mit dem beigelegten Ausdruck übereinstimmen. Bitte vermeiden Sie das Komprimieren der Dateien mit einem Packprogramm. Auf dem Etikett der Diskette müssen folgende Angaben vermerkt sein: Titel der Arbeit, Name des Erstautors, sowie verwendetes Betriebssystem und Software (Versionsnummer). Sowohl Disketten im Macintosh-Format als auch MS-DOS-formatierte Disketten werden akzeptiert. Speichern Sie den Text in dem vom Textverarbeitungsprogramm angebotenen Standardformat ab. Das bevorzugte Textverarbeitungsprogramm ist MS-Word. Dateien anderer verbreiteter Textverarbeitungsprogramme sowie ASCII-Formate können ebenfalls bearbeitet werden. Die Datei sollte keine Seitenlayout-Anweisungen, wie Hinweise zur Plazierung von Grafiken, enthalten. Bitte den Text linksbündig schreiben und keine Silbentrennungen durchführen. Erfassen Sie Ihren Text endlos, d.h. benutzen Sie harte Zeilenschaltungen (Return-Taste) nur am Ende eines Absatzes oder für Titel, Untertitel, etc. Bitte verwenden Sie **nur ein Format** (Normal) für die Erstellung des Textes. Dateien, die aufwendig formatiert sind, können nur unter Schwierigkeiten in das Satzprogramm übernommen werden. Zur Gliederung des Textes können Tabulatoren verwendet werden, Kopf- und Fußzeilen bitte vermeiden. Prüfen Sie, ob die folgenden Zeichen im Manuskript korrekt wiedergegeben sind: 1 (Eins) und l (Buchstabe), 0 (null) und O (Buchstabe), X (Buchstabe) und × (Malkreuz). Tabellen und Abbildungen bitte **nicht** in den Text integrieren, sondern als separate Dateien speichern (siehe auch «Abbildungen»). Es wird die Verwendung der Schriften Times und Symbol empfohlen.

Abbildungen

Illustrationen jeder Art sollten als separate Datei gespeichert werden. Die meisten der für die Erstellung der Abbildungen verwendeten Programme erlauben die Speicherung in verschiedenen Dateiformaten. TIFF, PostScript oder EPS werden bevorzugt. Die Abbildung sollte anhand des Dateinamens zugeordnet werden können. Zusätzlich müssen alle Abbildungen unbedingt als reproduktionsfähige Vorlagen mitgeliefert werden.

Literatur

Bitte beachten Sie für die Abfassung der Literatur die «Hinweise für Autoren». Verwenden Sie kein Komma nach dem Nachnamen und keine Punkte nach den Initialen. Nach Semikolon und Doppelpunkt darf kein Leerschlag eingefügt werden, *falsch:* Infusionsther Transfusionsmed 1998; 25: 160 – 3., *richtig:* Infusionsther Transfusionsmed 1998;25:160–163.

KARGER

Fax +49 761 4 52 07 14
E-mail Information@Karger.de
www.karger.com

Guidelines for Authors available at:
www.karger.com/journals/onk/onk_gl.htm